4-14

KEEP

Your Health...

IT

Your Body...

Your Energy...

UP

Your Strength...

THE POWER OF PRECISION MEDICINE TO CONQUER **LOW T** AND REVITALIZE YOUR LIFE

FLORENCE COMITE, MD

Foreword by ABRAHAM MORGENTALER, MD
associate clinical professor of urology, Harvard Medical School

RODALE.

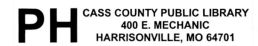

© 2013 by Florence Comite, MD

Foreword © 2013 by Abraham Morgentaler, MD

Rodale books may be purchased for business or promotional use or for special sales. For information, please write to:
Special Markets Department, Rodale Inc., 733 Third Avenue, New York, NY 10017

Printed in the United States of America

Rodale Inc. makes every effort to use acid-free ♾, recycled paper ♺.

Book design by Christopher Rhoads

Library of Congress Cataloging-in-Publication Data is on file with the publisher.

ISBN 978–1–60961–101–9   hardcover

Distributed to the trade by Macmillan

2   4   6   8   10   9   7   5   3   1   hardcover

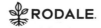

We inspire and enable people to improve their lives and the world around them.
rodalebooks.com

THIS BOOK IS DEDICATED TO MY MOTHER AND FATHER.

My understanding of health began with my mother. Her garden-raised, fresh cooked, natural food meals—nary a can in sight—kept my twin sister, my brother, me, and our host of friends healthy, happy, and . . . full. Vivid still, memories include her cold storage room, keeping garden vegetables fresh all year, and the years she pressed, with purple feet, garden grapes into wine.

My mother was also my earliest model of compassion. Daily, she carried fresh meals to elderly neighbors and received, in return, the pleasure that her food, conversation, and concern brought to them. The rhythms of her daily life, ingrained in my memory, help me to give as a physician. To listen. To serve. To hug. Together, these acts of compassion, the "therapeutic alliance," is quite possibly the most powerful healing tool a practitioner can offer.

My mother continues to garden at home in Pennsylvania, with my sister Harriet, the inheritor of the green thumb. Harriet is not only a master gardener, she is a busy dermatologist whose skilled hands have transformed lives.

From my father, we unconsciously absorbed the value of exercise. He took us outside as often as possible. He encouraged us in all sports, especially swimming. His three children were, no doubt, the only kids on the beach at Far Rockaway permitted to jump 20-foot, pre-storm waves. My brother Stephen absorbed our father's lessons best of all. Stephen, who, like Harriet, is a successful dermatologist, shepherded his children over the years through a universe of sports and outdoor activity.

Prior to emigrating to the United States, my parents faced loss, devastation, and near death in a war-ravaged Europe. They overcame great odds to create a loving home, live productive lives, and teach their children that "winning" is never the goal. Rather, it's about trying one's very best. Accordingly, their children try their very best to achieve loving homes and productive lives, to transmit the values of their parents to the next generation, and, as physicians, to help in the healing of the world.

CONTENTS

FOREWORD

On my first day of medical school, the dean made a welcoming speech to the incoming students: "Study hard while you're here," he said, "but be aware that within 10 years of graduating half of what you've learned will turn out to be incorrect."

How right he was! The shin bone may always be connected to the knee bone, but our knowledge, beliefs, and attitudes about health have changed beyond recognition from when my dean welcomed my fellow students and me 35 years ago. One key area that has changed is the critical role of hormones, especially testosterone in men, for maintaining our health.

My colleague Florence Comite, MD, is an endocrinologist who understands the importance of this forward thinking and has made it part of her life's work. It is not every day that one finds a kindred spirit trained in research-based medicine, yet with an interest in moving beyond the standard medical model of curing disease to helping men and women find their optimal health sweet spot. So, I am delighted to recommend *Keep It Up*, a marvelous guide to what men need to know about their bodies and their health in order to live long and to live well.

There are a great many health books out there, but this one is different. Medicine is changing, and what men are searching for is a guide that incorporates the latest insights with the best of established medical practice. This is such a book.

In these pages, Dr. Comite presents a forward-looking view on what it takes for men to live a healthy life, using what she has called *Precision Medicine* to get out ahead of disease and prevent it rather than waiting to treat it. Although the field of endocrinology (the part of medicine that deals with hormones) has a long and storied past, there is a new understanding of the nuances of hormones in men that is appreciated and advocated as yet by only a small vanguard of physicians. This change represents a true revolution in thought. I can attest to the critical importance of this approach from my own experience with the several thousand men who have walked through the doors of my own medical practice at Men's Health Boston. These men have gained an acute sense of vitality and renewed health with testosterone therapy as they had never thought possible before. In *Keep It Up*, Dr. Comite provides an insider's access to how an experienced, accomplished clinician thinks about some of the most common problems men face as they age, and what to do about them. And she offers a partnership with patients; that is the way good medicine should be practiced.

Many of the points and recommendations made in this book will be met with surprise and even scorn by the reader's regular physician. That's how it is when new information and beliefs meet old. My own experience bears this out.

As an undergraduate at Harvard University in the 1970s, I had performed research in lizards, finding that testosterone had critical functions on sexual behavior and acted as a brain hormone. During medical school and urology residency, I was taught almost nothing about testosterone. However, when I began my own urological practice in the late 1980s, I was curious about testosterone because of my prior research. I was surprised at how many of my patients had low testosterone levels. I was further surprised at how many reported feeling improved so quickly after I started them on testosterone therapy. Most had come to see me for sexual problems, yet when I saw them in follow-up, I was impressed by how often they would say something like, "My erections are better and so is my sex drive, but the thing I like best is how good I feel overall."

I soon began treating large numbers of men with testosterone, with excellent results. Many of my patients who did well had been told by their regular physicians that there was nothing wrong with them. "You're just getting older," their doctors would tell them. It wasn't true. These men had *low T*, as I called it. (I coined this term in the early 1990s to make it easier for discussions with patients and even some of my colleagues, who would feel uncomfortable when saying testosterone deficiency.) Their symptoms were real and caused by a hormone deficiency.

When I started doing this work, I didn't know a single physician treating men routinely with testosterone for sexual symptoms such as erectile dysfunction or diminished libido, and my colleagues regarded my work as bizarre. Soon I discovered a small cadre of like-minded physicians around the United States with similar interests in researching the benefits of testosterone, but our work was almost unknown. At scientific meetings I would often make the only presentation involving testosterone. Today, those same meetings devote entire days to testosterone research. How times have changed. Eventually, people do catch on. However, there is still much resistance among the medical community to the idea that low T is a legitimate and common condition that merits treatment.

What's important to know now is that testosterone is not all about sex, as is so often believed. As Dr. Comite discusses in detail, low T is also associated with symptoms of fatigue, depressed mood, reduced muscle mass and strength, and osteoporosis. Men with low T are at increased risk for developing diabetes, the metabolic syndrome (a set of conditions that predispose to cardiovascular risks, including obesity and high blood pressure), and atherosclerosis.

One of the great concerns about testosterone therapy has been the belief that higher testosterone levels cause an increased risk of prostate cancer. Fortunately, this turns out to be false. As I have reported in my research, the original concept was based on a single case in 1941, and numerous modern scientific studies have failed to show any connection between high testosterone levels and increased prostate cancer risk. In fact, in 2011 my colleagues and I published the first study of testosterone therapy in men with untreated low-grade prostate cancer, who were being monitored through active surveillance. Although the study was quite small, it was remarkable that not one of the men developed progression of their cancer after an average of 2½ years of testosterone treatment.

Today, men with prostate cancer regularly fly in to Boston from all over the world to ask me if they might be candidates for testosterone therapy. Offering testosterone therapy to these men was unthinkable a mere 10 years ago, when every medical student was taught that giving testosterone to a man with prostate cancer was akin to pouring gasoline on a fire. Why is this an important point? Because testosterone therapy not only helps these men feel better, it also helps these men live healthier lives by reducing their risk of disorders of aging, such as heart disease and diabetes.

Medicine is all about change, and Dr. Comite is at the leading edge of much of this change. She knows what men need in order to live optimally healthy lives. The traditional pillars of good health—nutrition and exercise—are still important, but to have true health and fitness, and to be on top of their game, men need to know about much more. In *Keep It Up*, Dr. Comite explores the importance of muscle, fat, blood sugar, insulin, diet, exercise, and overall metabolism. We are complex, biological, hormonal machines, but Dr. Comite makes it all understandable so that you can take charge of your health.

Congratulations on picking up this book. Now read it, and get armed to live life well.

—Abraham Morgentaler, MD, FACS
Associate clinical professor of urology, Harvard Medical School
Author of *Testosterone for Life* and *Why Men Fake It*
Founder and director of Men's Health Boston
menshealthboston.com

INTRODUCTION

Welcome to the century of personalization. Everything in our world is connected to you, the individual consumer. When you fire up your computer, your browser shows advertisements customized specifically for you based on what it has surmised about your likes by monitoring your search activity. Online stores will send an e-mail touting new ski goggles this week because last week you ordered a new snowboard. And iTunes offers artist suggestions based on your playlist. Soon, if Japanese inventors have their way, your car will recognize the highly personal imprint of your rear end—thanks to 350 sensors in the seat—making comfort adjustments and turning the engine on for only you to thwart car thieves.

Our 21st century medicine is becoming equally as personalized and integrated. I call this movement *Precision Medicine*. It's the simple idea that you are very unique, and as such, the decisions regarding your health care should be based on you, that unique individual, not some cohort of thousands of people who are similar but not quite *you*.

This futuristic style of medicine focuses on preventing disease long before an illness or disorder shows up as symptoms. How? By analyzing the most comprehensive and minute details about your body and your life—your daily choices, the foods you eat, the exercises you do, the controls and switches within your genes that turn on or off based on the lifestyle decisions you make day to day and year to year.

Mainstream medicine doesn't currently work this way. It's not at all individualized. Mainstream doctors practice what's called "evidence-based medicine," meaning they make a recommendation or choose a course of treatment based on evidence, that is, what clinical studies involving large groups of people have found to be prudent and effective.

But you are not a large group of people. You are you with a unique medical profile, family history, and lifestyle. You are different from everyone else in some way or other, even, yes, if you are an identical twin!

Precision Medicine takes this into account. Integrative doctors, like me, look at the whole person through the lens of a high-powered microscope, to use a science analogy. We want to know everything about your health and encourage you to become a student of your own physiology. Because with that knowledge comes the power to make meaningful alterations that truly prevent disease.

With this proactive, preventive health approach, you will be able to track your progress over time with a specificity that is unprecedented. It will reinforce the idea that you are an individual who is ultimately in control of his own health. Now, you may be thinking that you are a product of your genes and there's little you can do to influence the cards you were dealt (I thought so too once upon a time), but more and more evidence suggests this isn't the case. Even identical twins are different, and, believe it or not, all of us can alter the expression of our DNA. For example, if specific genetic markers reveal an increased risk of a heart attack, you can actually neutralize your risk by eating lots of fruits and vegetables.

This book is designed to teach you how to evaluate and quantify your own health and make key life-changing decisions that will dramatically increase your health span, the length of disease-free active, energetic living. You know your body better than anyone. You are the writer of your own story. In these pages, you'll meet men just like you who are enjoying the benefits of good health because they saw where their stories were headed and they took charge of their bodies in time to write new chapters of their lives. Here is one of these men:

It seemed to have happened overnight. I hit 40 and, boom, my battery was drained. I just felt tired and lousy. I'm in a competitive field—I work for an international government agency—and it requires some type A motivation and effort, so this was a real problem. I asked my doctor to test my testosterone level. "I bet it's low," I offered. My doctor said, "No, no, no, you don't need to worry about hormones. Low T is normal as you age."

It took me a while to convince him, but he finally tested me. My levels were very low. "But hormone levels fluctuate throughout the day," he told me, "and stress affects them." What he could do was test my testosterone over a longer period of time when my life wasn't stressful. Yeah, right. Like that's going to happen. Stress is the norm for me. I travel regularly to third world countries, real hot spots complete with gunfire and kidnappings. I spent a year and a half in Iraq. So the low-stress thing is never going to happen, and I didn't know where to turn for help until I found an endocrinologist named Florence Comite.

Dr. Comite was convinced that improving my diet and raising my testosterone level would help. She gave me a total makeover strategy: diet plan, exercise, supplements, hormone therapy, and more, but here's the thing: I didn't follow the plan. I took the medications and supplements, used what she gave me to boost my testosterone, but when it came to the exercise and diet, I just didn't do the work. Six months later, I'm back in her office, and she can see in my body and in the lab data that I'm not doing everything she said to do.

"Look at your numbers," she said. "Your body is primed to take advantage of all this. You're in the sweet spot. Your gains will be huge, but you have to follow through."

That motivated me to follow the program. Next thing I know, my pants don't fit anymore. Within 6 months, I lost 16 pounds of fat and gained 24 pounds of muscle. My body fat composition improved, decreasing by almost 10 percent to 18. My muscle, my attitude, my stamina, and my overall health are like they were in my twenties. I never thought it would be possible.

—**Kirk Hansen,** age 49, government official

Remember how it used to be? In your twenties, you had a much more intense sex drive, you were ready to do battle at any meeting, whenever necessary, and you still had energy to spare to go out after work or play a pickup game of basketball with your buddies. You could burn off a few pounds in a weekend. You could eat almost anything you wanted and not gain weight. You could run to your heart's content and not feel it in your knees. You could party on a weeknight and still get through a tough day at the office. There was nothing you couldn't accomplish. You felt certain. You felt decisive. You felt invincible.

These days you may be feeling a bit different. Maybe you're hungering for those glory days, or perhaps you're just hoping to have enough energy to make it through the afternoons at work. That feeling of toughness has softened into apathy, a weary acceptance of the passing years. As the understanding of your own mortality deepens—the wrinkles on your face, the inches around your waist, the nagging health problems, all supporting evidence that, yes, you aren't in your twenties (or thirties) anymore—perhaps you don't even care. But there's a way to get you back to that sweet spot. It's not gone for good. You can have that quality of life again. You are *not* helplessly sliding into old age. You *can* get back to the top of your game; you *can* have the energy, the drive, and even the health of a younger you. It's *possible*.

As an endocrinologist who has worked predominantly with men in recent years, I've witnessed major turnarounds in the health of hundreds of men—the reversal of type 2 diabetes and cardiovascular disease, even the repair of heart tissue damaged by heart attack. I've seen men go from having no sex drive to asking me to dial it back a bit because their wives are exhausted from all the attention. I've had 50-year-old patients who looked 10 years younger within a year; men who were overweight and out of shape who became highly energetic and seriously sculpted; athletes who felt sidelined who were able to fulfill youthful dreams of playing their favorite sport again, now at a higher level than they ever thought possible. I am going to help you accomplish the same things my patients have accomplished. I'll give you the tools and guidance you need so that you can become the healthiest version of you, enjoying life to the fullest until the last moment.

Losing your game is not inevitable. What I'm proposing for you is what I call Precision Medicine, a strategic approach to disease prevention that is based on real cutting-edge science and clinical evidence. You can do a 180 and retrieve your energy, strength, libido, erectile function, mental clarity, and more, just like you had when you were a younger man starting out in life.

WHY YOU'RE FEELING THE WAY YOU DO NOW

I'll spare you the clichés of the most obvious symptoms of an aging man. It's time for a new understanding of what's happening at this moment so that we can develop a more productive response to the semiconscious feelings of despair that drive some men toward the destructive midlife crises. This is what I hear from men: *I don't feel so great anymore. I'm not at the top of my game at home or at work. My kids are running me ragged. Working out doesn't work anymore. I want to feel strong and energetic again, but nothing I do seems to work. I feel like I'm turning into my father and slowing down.*

Well, you're not stuck; downward is not the only direction you can go. There is a physiological explanation for how you're feeling, and you can do something about it. You can change how you look and feel by taking ownership of your health.

ENTER ANDROPAUSE

What's causing you to feel the way you do has a medical name: andropause. It's derived from the Greek *andros* (man) and *pauses* (cessation).

Like menopause in women, andropause is a gradual hormonal change that occurs naturally in your body over the course of a decade or more. Beginning in your thirties, your body starts to slow its production of male hormones, primarily testosterone, the main sex hormone and the "rocket fuel" that has powered your health, energy, sexuality, and state of mind for most of your life. Testosterone production continues to decline in your forties and fifties. By age 65, more than 75 percent of men have experienced andropause, the most significant measurable indicator being low testosterone, or "low T."

You've likely seen the low-T commercials on TV during ball games, advertising testosterone gels and creams. Andropause and low T are gaining media attention, and doctors, too, are starting to recognize symptoms in their patients when only a few years ago most physicians did not believe there was a menopause equivalent in males. The relationship between your hormones and the way your body functions is rather linear; unlike in women, though, hormonal decline in men is subtle and often undetectable from day to day, month to month, even year to year. Still, you can recognize it if you know what to look for. As testosterone diminishes, you feel the reduction in lean muscle, it becomes harder to lose fat, especially around the middle, and you put on weight faster. The abdominal fat tends to be dangerous visceral fat—the kind that forms on your organs and pushes out a belly that feels hard and solid and increases your chances for having a heart attack. Mentally, you're not as clear as you once were. You're dealing with lethargy, low libido, insomnia, mood changes, lack of clarity, listlessness, and more. Yes, all those complaints that many people think are natural side effects of aging. One of the most noticeable signs of low testosterone is the loss of those morning erections that used to salute the start of your day. You begin to lose your drive, your tenacity, your focus, and your competitiveness. Again, these changes don't occur overnight; often they fly under your radar, a surreptitious entrance. You'll cross a threshold, which is different for everyone, and you may not be aware there's a problem until your doctor says you're a prediabetic, or you have a heart attack. All of a sudden, it's real for you: You're aging. You have a disease that once applied only to your grandfather, or maybe your father, not to you. It's been brewing for years—you've either ignored the insidious signals or explained them away: *Work is tough. I'm tired. I'm traveling a lot. My wife and I have been together for a long time, and things aren't as exciting as they used to be, but we're okay. Sex isn't as important now. Besides, we're busy with the kids.*

This is the norm, but it doesn't have to be this way.

It seems inevitable that your health declines as the years pass. Peak health is typically in synchrony with your best reproductive years, your late twenties. After all, nature didn't intend for us to reproduce for the rest of our lives. However, because medical knowledge is expanding so rapidly, we don't have to sit back and accept nature's plan; we don't have to give up or give in. We can intervene. You can take advantage of new insights and technologies to evaluate your state of health and take charge of the rest of your life so as to prevent the diseases that put the face on what we see as aging.

Medical science is starting to see the relationship between the shifts in your hormones and what you're feeling. We don't understand what we don't know. I say this a lot, and it's true. Clinical studies are (just) beginning to show correlations between the drop in testosterone and the onset of the disorders of aging like heart disease, cancer, diabetes, kidney disease, and more.

Modern medical care focuses on treating your major organs—your heart, lungs, and digestive system—and has failed to recognize that changes in hormones play a significant role in your entire body. And although we recognize that hormones impact adolescents as they go through puberty, until recently we haven't given hormones the same consideration as we age. We can't look at organs or even organ systems in isolation anymore. In medical school, I was trained to examine organ systems while not necessarily acknowledging them as communicating entities. Hormones are the messengers that allow the various systems to work synergistically to carry out your body's processes in an ideal setting. If our hormones fail to work in an optimal manner, you can imagine what happens to us as a whole. Through more than 30 years of clinical research and patient care, I've learned how to listen to the orchestra, the separate sections, and singling out individual instruments as appropriate. There's a dialogue that's going on between all your parts, each interacting and influencing every other element in the highly complex ecosystem that is the human body. Understanding that dialogue, which is taking place on the cellular level, is part of the future of medicine. I predict that the practices I will describe on these pages will be the standard of health care within 20 years. But you don't have to wait that long. You can benefit now by learning much more about your body and how it's changing, and by taking personal responsibility for its optimal performance.

FATHER KNOWS BEST

In medical school, I was taught the foundation of health and disease concepts and was given the tools and the skills to question the validity of evidence and research. That was important, yet it was watching my father age that opened my eyes to the possibilities of preventive maintenance. Dad was ahead of his time—he was passionate about maintaining his strength, as well as preventing health problems by working out and watching his diet. He exercised religiously into his nineties and lived a healthy life right up to the end.

Dad wasn't just dedicated to keeping himself healthy. He had an insatiable curiosity about how he could do things better, what he could learn, what more he could do. As I evolved as a doctor, he would ask me the same set of questions: *How do I stay healthy? What should I eat? What should I do?* Every time I began a new field of study in medicine, he'd ask me again. So I kept looking for more answers—for my father, myself, and everyone else.

When I was younger, I was frustrated with our medical system as I saw it. I was trained traditionally in diagnosing and managing disease, as a reactive approach, after a disorder had already showed up waving a red flag and announcing, "I'm bad news." Med school emphasized figuring out the diagnosis when a patient presented by putting together a "differential," that is, listing, in descending order, the most likely reasons that would explain a set of symptoms. We were, and still are, mostly focused on stamping out disease, putting out fires, and helping sick people. These are all noble causes, but it seemed clear to me that if you could start the intervention *before* symptoms arose, you could accomplish much more. You might even be able to keep people from getting so sick in the first place.

The sad truth is that often doctors don't have enough time to educate you on all the details they might see. Or, at your annual checkup (you are going every year or so, I hope), your "slightly" high blood sugar level or "borderline" cholesterol lab results are minimized, perhaps to avoid frightening you. It takes time for a thorough analysis that will expose imbalance in your system early on. Our traditional course of medical delivery is intervention that waits for disease to appear, symptoms to be obvious, signs to be palpable, labs to be grossly out of range. Instead of looking at the signals of the disorders of aging in our thirties, forties, and fifties, we—and particularly men—frequently wait until the chest pain occurs or we develop a persistent cough or an infection that doesn't heal.

My father's questions about how to stay healthy kept bringing me back to why I wanted to be a doctor in the first place: to keep my patients healthy for as long as possible, to *prevent* disease. My father's life choices prompted me to find out more about how to accomplish that goal and ultimately led me to change the way I thought about medicine and healing individuals.

I want to invert the model and identify risk before your doctor is forced to take heroic and immediate action—in order to prevent the truck that nobody saw from plowing you down in the form of a heart attack, diabetes, cancer, or kidney disease. That metaphorical truck didn't just appear out of nowhere. It started its journey toward you hundreds of miles away. It might have begun a generation or two before you were standing at that critical intersection. That accident waiting to happen was possibly laced into your DNA and brought about by lifestyle. Yet, mainstream medicine is set up only to intervene when the truck is barreling down on you—when the threat of disease is looming and possibly reversible only through aggressive intervention. But you can redirect the truck on to a new route by paying attention to yourself, gaining a deeper understanding of how your genetics and lifestyle choices impact you. That's the kind of medicine I want to practice. I want to improve whole lives rather than fix diseased parts. I want to help people invest in their health as active participants rather than as consumers of medications. Fortunately, the tools and the knowledge to do that are here, and more are just on the horizon.

The other thing I learned from my father is that there is a direct relationship between how well you know yourself—which means being totally honest with yourself about how you eat, act, think, and live—and the kind of care you are able to get. When I would push him to go to a doctor before he was ready, he would say to me, "What is he going to tell me that I don't already know? I live in my body. I know what it feels like. I keep a record of it. I will know when it's time to go see the doctor." He was pretty much right every time.

You too can become clued in about the state of your body. You will gather the details of your habits, your health, your family's medical history, and combine this with the numbers from your lab data. Observation and tracking changes over time is the key, and I give you the tools so that you can build the same personalized health portfolio that I help my patients create. You read bank statements and quarterly reports all the time. You understand what the numbers mean and you know how to make adjustments to turn around situations that are going in the wrong direction. What you'll do as you read this book is similar. You'll learn to read your own numbers—everything from body composition to the results of your blood work—just like you read financial statements. You'll see within your own lab test results where you're moving in the right direction and where you need to focus more. Knowledge is power, and with the right medical wisdom and guidance to help you interpret the data and implement solutions, you will have the best foundation possible for a long and vibrant life.

THE BIG PROMISE:
YOU CAN FEEL 25 AGAIN!

We all get older. Chronological aging is unavoidable. But how you age is well within your control. By taking direct, tangible, proactive steps, any man, at virtually any age, can return to prime physical condition, restore energy, sharpen his mind, revive his sex drive, and, believe it or not, regain the metabolic and hormonal functioning of a 25-year-old. That's right. Biologically, you can be 25 again.

You can turn back the clock. Reclaiming the body and the physical and mental performance of a younger you is absolutely possible. I see it every day in my patients from around the world and have hundreds of success stories to prove it. In this book, you will meet some of those men who have turned their health around. There's also real research and real science to back up this new aggressive, proactive approach to health. Here's what you can expect.

- All the symptoms that you've been grappling with for years will likely improve within months, maybe weeks. The initial changes that happen very quickly are in those nagging issues that you think are part of daily life. For example, can't go without your 3:00 p.m. nap, and your golf game is down to 9 holes instead of 18? Do you have difficulty getting an erection? You can expect to turn all these around in a short time. Shifts can happen that are very up front and very immediate. If you choose to pay attention to your exercise, diet, and other habits, change is not just possible, it's probable.

- With time, you will begin to recognize and appreciate the cause and effect of the positive changes you make. If you're a prediabetic or diabetic, you'll be able to reverse that. If you have high cholesterol, you will see how lifestyle changes will bring those numbers down. You will see tangible, measureable results and these will be reflected in your precision health analysis. You'll lose weight and need to buy new clothes that fit. You'll have more energy. You'll see your muscles through your T-shirt. All the superficial stuff of New Year's resolutions and reality

TV shows will improve. More importantly, through sleep, stress reduction, diet, exercise, key medications, and supplements, you will begin remodeling yourself from the inside out, becoming healthier and even feeling younger.

I get great satisfaction from seeing my patients live the life they want, actually getting more energetic, confident, stronger, and more active with each birthday. Given the fact that the average life expectancy of a man has grown significantly over the past 50 years, you need to focus on extending your personal *health span* in order to keep up with your extended *life span*. Healthy longevity means being vibrant, active, happy, and pain free well into your nineties. It's within your power to maintain and even improve your well-being for as long as possible. You want to live life to its fullest as you did in the prime of your life. I want you to keep your confidence, energy, drive, power, ambition, and control. Together we can ensure your good health for years to come.

[Many of my patients have graciously allowed me to use their personal stories as examples in this book. Some have given permission to use their full names, while others have chosen to remain anonymous and use a pseudonym. I am grateful to them all for sharing their testimonials in the hope of helping other men. –FC]

CHAPTER 1

THE GAME IS CHANGING

Can your body keep up with what modern culture expects of it as the decades pass?

The realization that I wasn't what I used to be came a couple years ago when I was in the Congo tromping through the jungle. I'm a photographer. Jane Goodall was there, and she's 77 and kicking the [crap] out of the entire crew. All these guys couldn't keep up with her. Throughout my career, I'd always been the strongest guy on my crew. I'd be in Dubai running up a sand dune leaving my younger assistants in the dust. But suddenly that was over for me. I'd lost that. I could feel myself failing. It was horrible. When I got my blood work back from Dr. Comite, my cortisol [stress hormone] levels surprised me. I know what it feels like to be stressed out, but I'd never seen being stressed out illustrated as a number before, chemically. My testosterone levels were low, of course, and whatever improvements I could make to my physical

1

infrastructure through hormone treatment and exercise was my primary concern. I didn't just want to be better. I wanted to be optimal. I'm competing with the best in the world.

I felt results right away. I had more energy, and now Dr. Comite tells me that I've essentially reversed the aging process in most of my measurable tests. Travel is still the biggest obstacle for me. I avoid the junk foods that are easily accessible, like in hotel mini-bars. Also, I've never had a steady, normal schedule. In my work, I have to keep a second suitcase packed at all times because I don't know when or where I'm going next. So I work very hard to eat right and stay on the program no matter where I am. I rededicated myself to the good things I had already been doing while including the newer ideas from Dr. Comite and her staff, such as adding intervals to my workouts. My God, has that helped me! I am now out on a shoot and not even feeling it.

–VINCENT M., age 53, photographer

The baby boomers have forever changed what a 40-year-old looks like and what he can do with his body. The transformation began in the 1980s, when many people started exercising more and eating better. They also were starting their families later in life. All this got pushed up against the wall of the body's natural slowdown, and the health impact became obvious. It used to be you might live into your fifties, dying from the disorders of aging instead of surviving to deal with their complications. Today, you'll likely live into your eighties, so now the question becomes, *How well will you live those added years? How will you sustain health beyond your peak?* If life begins at 40, as the saying goes, then we need to make sure the body can keep up.

Here's the problem: Countless men hitting their forties come into my office and tell me that everything seems like it's just grinding down—that their best years are over. If you're feeling that way, and facing four more decades of life, that has serious implications.

Growing older in the current medical climate isn't pretty. It's full of knees that don't work, beer guts that persist even after you stop drinking, a disappearing sex drive, and a steadily weakening of body and mind until some debilitating disease takes you out. It doesn't seem fair or practical. Our quality of life is suffering, and our health care system is crashing because it wastes billions to manage chronic disorders year after year. We have extension of life but not extension of health. I don't want to see folks in the last one, two, three, or even four decades of life having few choices in how they live except to cater to the complications of avoidable diseases.

You will likely live longer thanks to modern medicine, and you too can be like my dad and live to see your nineties. If you take action now, you can age in good health like my father fortunately did. He took the initiative to eat right and exercise. He monitored his health and challenged himself to improve in a way that people usually don't do on their own. My father was the first person to shape my ideas on Precision Medicine. Knowing yourself and taking ownership of your health will help you keep going strong physically, mentally, and socially. Doctors may not always ask the right questions, so it pays to be aware as Livingston Miller's story illustrates.

I'm a trainer, so I eat right and I stay in shape. I've appeared in ads all over New York City for a gym, advertised as the picture of health. I was training Dr. Comite and talked to her about some of the problems I was having—getting dizzy periodically, feeling thirsty all the time, and fainting. I was drinking a lot of fluid and urinating so much that I cut back on water. When I had gone to another doctor, he thought I was dehydrated because of my intense physical activity. He wasn't alarmed by my elevated blood sugar either because I ate five meals a day. I even passed out a few times and was brought to the ER. There, they had no idea what was wrong with me, even with multiple tests, CAT scans, too. My symptoms persisted, and Dr. Comite was hearing my frustration. After another episode when I passed out just after snacking on a protein bar at the end of a long day of golf, I told Dr. Comite, and she got me evaluated right away. When the lab test results came back, I was in for the shock of my life. I was a diabetic. Then I underwent a VO_2 assessment, and the findings caused her to suspect that I had had a silent heart attack sometime in the past. Next I underwent a nuclear stress test, which confirmed the muscle damage in the inferior portion of my heart. My cholesterol was 240. I got onto her program, lost 20 pounds, and turned the diabetes around completely with supplements and eating the right food at the right times. I got my cholesterol down and have been repairing the damage from the heart attack.

—LIVINGSTON MILLER, age 59, personal trainer

Livingston's symptoms were classic signs of diabetes. Before I brought him in for testing, I asked him, "Who in your family has diabetes?" His response: "Everyone." That didn't surprise me, and it indicated that I was on the right track. After I ran his blood work and saw his sugar metabolism numbers (see his hemoglobin A1c shown on page 237), my hunch was confirmed. If he had been asked about his family history earlier, the other doctor might not have glossed over his high blood sugar. If doctors had more time with patients, we could get to know them. By asking the right questions, we would be better able to identify such warning signs. That's why you have to know your family's health history and your own health data, a process I'll help guide you through in this book. With this knowledge, you'll be the one to optimize your own health and ensure the quality of your life at any age.

Livingston has done a health 180. What did he change? He's getting adequate sleep; he's practicing stress reduction; he's training properly for his body—significantly cutting back on the resistance training, replacing it with more cardio. He's mostly eating the right food regularly throughout the day and is drinking less wine too; he's taking supplements and even some medications for balance. I have him on a statin for his cholesterol because I want to see it lower than the 180 milligrams per deciliter (mg/dL) he has been able to attain with lifestyle changes. I've also started him on testosterone, which has benefited his metabolism. For Livingston, it's *game on*. Now he has the chance to keep his edge for the rest of his life. If he stays on track, he will likely be in good health for decades to come, despite having hit a rocky patch in his late forties.

But imagine if Livingston's disorders of aging—heart disease and diabetes—had gone undetected. His future might have looked as it does for many seniors facing constant hospitalizations, with limited mobility and mental faculties. I don't want this to be the way anyone lives their last years. And it doesn't have to be.

I've been a doctor for 36 years. I studied and taught medicine at Yale Medical School at Yale University, and I've been fortunate to work with some of the brightest minds in the medical world. I'm an endocrinologist,

Which 84-Year-Old Do You Want to Be?

I've shrunk to about 100 pounds. I have diabetes and I'm in the hospital after breaking my second hip. I was home for only 3 weeks after the repair of my first hip fracture. My wife and son are by my bedside constantly, and I'm not able to eat much. I'm failing fast, and I feel I'm helpless. After being strong all my life, I never thought I could become so frail.

—SAM, retired electrician

I founded an investment banking firm over 40 years ago, and I never imagined that I would stop working. I wanted to be able to get into the office at least twice a week; still, even that was becoming impossible. It was pretty depressing to feel incapacitated. My available testosterone level was 14, and I was told that was less than you'd find in a boy, not even a teen. I started on testosterone and several supplements, including DHEA (dehydroepiandrosterone), vitamin D, coenzyme Q10. Within a few weeks, I'm not only at the office every day, I'm in the gym every day too. I even wake up with erections. I hadn't seen that action for years! I feel stronger, with more energy. My whole attitude has changed.

—GEORGE, investment banker

which means I look at communication throughout the body through the interaction of hormones and proteins, these agents in essence determining much of how we think and feel every day and over the course of our lives.

I've had the opportunity to study the human body in all its stages: in utero; early childhood; school-age years; the teenage years, when hormaonal surges trigger puberty; the twenties, when the body reaches its physiological and reproductive peak; the thirties, when hormone production begins to shift and dial back; the forties, when physiological and reproductive challenges usually become noticeable; the fifties, when health and disease consequences may develop, the product of unchecked disorders of aging; and the sixties, seventies, and so on.

The usual model has been to try to repair the body's malfunctioning systems and parts with medicine, which commonly shuts down any remaining functionality, creating a lifelong dependency on pharmaceauticals. When you replace thyroid hormone, for example, the thyroid gland stops working, and you are likely to need alternative sources of thyroid hormones for the rest of your life. My passion has been to find a way to help the body regain balance naturally, when possible, to restart sluggish metabolic function while triggering optimal hormonal activity. Lifestyle factors like sleep, stress, sex, nutrition, and exercise all impact the body's operation.

I've done clinical research at both Yale and the National Institutes of Health (NIH) that required thinking about how to help the body do a better job of taking care of itself when something isn't functioning well. My early focus was on pediatrics, specifically puberty that occurs too early, and later I helped develop Women's Health at Yale. My role, at that point, was to serve as a consultant; often many patients were interested in participating in my research trials on hormonal function once they met me. I wasn't a primary care doctor but the person a specialist conferred with when a patient was not making progress, a diagnosis was proving difficult to determine, or alternative management approaches were needed. A gynecologist might send her patient to me, for instance. I would assess the patient's health, make a diagnosis, then make recommendations, some of which may have derived from my research efforts. I acted as a tertiary consultant in many cases in that I conferred with specialists, but I didn't replace them or the primary physicians.

In the 1980s, I began to hear many stories that sounded similar. Women would tell me that they didn't know what was happening to their bodies. They felt lethargic, anxious, and generally just not like themselves. Some of these women were medical researchers and writers who had access to the literature, and they still didn't really know what was wrong. They would tell me: "Nobody seems to be able to answer my questions. I was told it's all in my head." Diagnoses were anything but physical: often empty-nest syndrome, depression, or something similar. Many of these women were given prescriptions for diazepam (Valium) or chlordiazepoxide (Librium). They were told to adopt a puppy. They were told to get over it. These women, baby boomers who were starting to feel the effects of aging, considered these answers unacceptable and kept searching for different solutions.

What became clear to me was that these women weren't being taken seriously and they weren't going to stay silent. They were not like their parents, who would rarely challenge their physician. Plus, they were part of the sandwich generation, raising a family yet also largely responsible for the care of their aging parents, who often were in poor health. They were concerned about following in the same path, adding burdens for their own children in the future.

As an endocrinologist, I knew that their hormones were in transition, declining each year. The cascade was producing a physiological change that was fundamentally transforming their bodies and shaping their minds, attitudes, and energy. Then it clicked: This time in life—menopause, for women—was an unwinding of what had begun to wind up in puberty. This epiphany led me to start down the road of appreciating how we can optimize the body's function to prevent the downward slide that we had assumed was inevitable with age. We could do it by bolstering the body's ability to regain hormonal balance. And if this was true for women, it was probably true for men as well.

Unexpectedly to me, the number one complaint I heard from women over 40 was actually not about their own health or the fact that they had put on a few pounds. It was about the failing health of their husband or male partner—their man's lack of energy, his weakening of libido. What's more, women were not only complaining about their men, they were losing interest in their partners because of it. The failing health of their husbands was the number one reason many women cited for having affairs.

The more I studied men over 40, the more I began to see a pattern of change for them, similar to menopause in women. Most of the men I was seeing had hit the same wall. They were exercising but getting no results. Recovering from workouts or injuries was becoming harder. They were eating right and still gaining weight, even the competitive athletes. For many men, their sex drive was disappearing. They didn't have the energy to do anything outside of work. And they couldn't keep up at work in the same way as they had previously. Their enthusiasm for any or all of their passions was limited. Many of them were trying to do everything they thought would give them a long and healthy life, but they were feeling worn out.

I wanted to understand why they were having these issues and figure out how to improve their quality of life. I was captivated by the developing field of andrology. I was particularly interested in how the brain's hypothalamus and pituitary signaled the testes and the gonads to produce testosterone (T)—a hormone that directly impacts a man's metabolism, muscles, and major organs.

What I knew was that I didn't know enough. I had to dig for more information, especially about men's experiences. Years went by and I couldn't find an organized field of study geared toward protecting the health and energy of men as we were doing for women. In 1991, the NIH in Bethesda, Maryland, had established the Office on Women's Health; no comparable office exists for men almost 25 years later. Throughout my tenure as a faculty member at Yale, I held a triple appointment in the departments of internal medicine, pediatrics, and gynecology. Andrology was conspicuously absent. In fact, while gynecology departments exist in every academic medical center, the few select andrology departments primarily focus on male infertility. More recently, several medical universities have launched health centers for men. Still, it is a field of medicine that isn't formally defined, nor is training readily available. Andrology is still in its inception.

It is clear that hormones are as important to men as they are to women. So why were men being overlooked? Not surprisingly, there have always been inequities between the sexes in terms of health care and research. Most research in men, in contrast to that in women, has been geared toward studying the major organs, like the heart, without focusing on metabolism and hormones or overall health. Men generally have not sought out answers to issues related to aging. You will see that we have begun to realize that heart disease (particularly the risk of having a heart attack) is associated with erectile dysfunction, which I will explain in more detail in Chapter 6. Many doctors still do not know about or agree with the data that has been published in renowned journals such as the *American Journal of Cardiology* or the *Journal of Urology*.

HOW YOUR BODY IS CHANGING

If you zoom out to the 30,000-foot view, you can see the pattern of change over your lifetime. Recall when you were a very young man, almost a kid. Think back to how you fought for what you wanted in your twenties and early thirties. Do you have that kind of energy and drive in your forties? Making this comparison will help you get a better sense of the contrast between where you were then and where you are now. You more than likely had more testosterone back then, and that helped you power through.

Let's look at how men's bodies change over the decades. The word "individual" is an important one here. Remember puberty? Some boys hit it at 11, some at 13, and some even later, at age 16 or 17. By the end of high school, almost everyone has experienced similar maturation changes to some degree. That's what you need to keep in mind through-out this journey: Aging is fiercely individual, yet inevitably universal.

THE TWENTIES

If you're a baseball fan—and I love the Yankees—you may know the conventional wisdom that says most players peak during their age-27 season. I believe this might be an official baseball fact as far as batting or pitching stats go, barring the illegal use of steroids over the past few decades. What you may not have known is that general medical science backs up this assumption: Men are at their peak around their middle to late twenties, depending on the individual.

Testosterone levels are generally at their highest too. Bone foundation and muscle strength peak at this time as well because of the more abundant T. You feel at the top of your game with respect to virility, physical performance, and energy. You feel confident and invulnerable. This feeling is not just a psychological state; it is directly influenced by your hormones, by the strength of your endocrine system and the amount of testosterone you have circulating through your body.

THE THIRTIES

As you march through your thirties, you may or may not notice some day-to-day changes such as the following:

- You can't party all night on a Tuesday and be fully alert and ready to go to work Wednesday morning.

- Even if you don't party, you can't burn the candle at both ends. Long hours at the office, poor sleep, and stress take a toll on your performance, unlike a decade earlier. You used to be able to work 12- or 15-hour days without stopping on the weekends. Now, if you try to push straight through, your thinking becomes fuzzy. You may find yourself nodding off at your desk or even in the middle of a meeting.

- When you work out, it's not as productive. You can't increase stamina. You used to notice results after a week or two, but now the time at the gym isn't having much impact. You're trying new exercises but not putting on muscle. When you overdo it, it takes a few days, even a week, before you can get back to exercising because your body just hurts too much.

- Your body isn't as taut as it used to be, and that's because you are losing lean muscle mass—the main protection for your bones and your immune system. Decline in lean muscle mass accelerates with every passing year unless you take action to reverse it.

- When you want to shed weight, it's a bit tougher. It used to be you could knock off 5 pounds after a couple of long runs or by cutting back on food for a few days. Not anymore. No matter what you do, you seem to keep gaining weight.

- You aren't as hungry as you used to be. And I don't mean for food. I'm talking about everything you lusted after: achievement, money, sex, competition. The edge isn't as sharp. The drive just isn't there.

THE FORTIES AND BEYOND

Now is when you start seeing the real visual signs of aging: You're needing reading glasses when you had perfect vision before; you grow hair everywhere, except your head; you develop skin tags, jowls, a wrinkled neck, and laugh lines. Your morning puffy eyes stay that way all day. Your skin is dry and wrinkled because it becomes thinner with less elasticity and collagen as you age. You've got more visible spider veins in your legs, as venous valves become less competent in driving blood back up to the heart. You've got bluish streaks on your face and nose, typically due to excess alcohol (think W. C. Fields) or other underlying triggers (more common in fair-skinned folks with rosacea). All of these things no longer resolve as easily as in your youth. And there's more:

- You are experiencing daily aches and pains in body parts you didn't even know you had.

- Your knees hurt after a run or when you climb up a few flights of stairs while carrying a heavy computer case.

- You start wearing your pants lower on your torso to accommodate the overhanging belly. Even when you diet and drastically cut back on calorie consumption, the weight doesn't come off. If you do lose a few pounds, it quickly comes back.

- You see serious and even fatal diseases in people who are in your age bracket. You may even know a close friend or colleague who has suffered a fatal heart attack.

- You blank out on a co-worker's name, someone you see every day. You can't recall memorized facts. In fact, you can't even memorize facts anymore.

- If you don't write it down when someone tells you something in the hallway, you won't remember it by the time you get back to your desk. Your short-term memory is not as dependable as it used to be, and it becomes even less reliable when you are worried or under stress. You find yourself wondering where you've left your reading glasses or end up squinting to read.

- Traveling beats you up. You can't take a red-eye and then head straight for the office after a quick shower. Instead, you need to sleep for a few hours, so you find a way to work from home.

- Your workouts just aren't working out anymore. You don't get to the gym as often because there isn't enough time. When you do go, generally you don't see much in terms of results. It may take a while to recover from a tough training session. Exercising feels like a waste of time.

- You don't get morning erections like when you were 25. Testosterone production has significantly slowed down, this process having begun for most men in their early-to-mid thirties. Your brain is already feeling the effect of receding levels of testosterone, as the cells responsible for turning you on are turning off. Your libido is not surging as it did in the past.

- Even if you get some morning erections and still have a fairly strong libido, you're generally not checking out every object of sexual interest on the street. You've begun to accept your diminished sexual drive and activity, like this patient of mine.

"I used to be able to do it every day, but my partner doesn't really want much anymore, so I'm not worried about it."

And another patient who explained:

"We've been together a long time. Things aren't as exciting in our marriage as they used to be, and I'm really stressed about work, so I'm just not as interested in sex as I used to be. Plus, the kids end up in our bed during the night."

They may be right. These reasons do contribute to a slowdown in sexual activity. However, infrequent morning erections and other physical signs are not completely under your conscious control. Beneath the surface, the physiological mechanisms that lead to desire, erections, and more are less active, inevitably slowing you down.

As you move past 45, the decline accelerates. At that age, more men will be noticing more symptoms. Put ten 35-year-olds together in a room, and maybe 1 or 2 of them will notice that they aren't quite as energetic as they used to be. When that same group hits 40, it might be half of them. At 50, it'll be 8 out of 10. By the time they hit 55 or 60, it's likely all 10.

WHY IS THIS HAPPENING TO ME?

Hormonal levels vary dramatically throughout life, and even over the course of an hour, depending on maturation and the individual. They increase and decrease as the hypothalamus and the pituitary respond to alterations in circulating hormones and proteins. Hormones—whether testosterone, thyroid, insulin, cortisol (the stress hormone), or any number of others—affect your drive, energy, attitude, and emotion. They influence every system in your body, regulating how you metabolize food; how your arteries expand to circulate blood; how your brain functions; how you focus; whether you want to eat, have sex, sleep, or exercise. As hormones diminish along with the signals from the brain to produce them, you begin to slow down.

When the hypothalamus and pituitary sense a downturn in the circulation of testosterone, for example, this should trigger the release of brain hormones that stimulate the testicles to ramp up production of testosterone. The specific brain hormones include gonadotropin releasing hormone (abbreviated GnRH), which is released by the hypothalamus, and luteinizing hormone (abbreviated LH), released by the pituitary. They act to control the production of testosterone in synchrony. This response system in your body that triggers the manufacture and release of hormones is a negative feedback loop. When this loop is functioning at its best, the body gets enough testosterone to bind to receptors on the various organs that require it.

In the bodies of men as they hit their thirties and forties, testosterone falls approximately 1 to 3 percent each year. Men entering their forties may have levels that are too low to maintain peak metabolic function. This leads to decreased muscle mass, a gain in fat (especially in the belly), less energy, sapped libido, erectile dysfunction, brain fog, and more. Not all symptoms occur in all men, of course. Sleep deprivation, stress, nutrition, exercise, genetics factors, and personal health and family relationships can all influence how you experience those symptoms, which range from mild to severe.

Think of your brain like a baseball coach who is out in left field, literally. It's not paying attention to the decrease in testosterone. Execution is lacking, yet the coach (your brain) keeps ignoring messages to send in the designated hitters GnRH and LH to stimulate the production of testosterone by the testes. Something's definitely going wrong here; your brain has been desensitized to these lower levels of testosterone. Scientists don't yet know why, but it's the reality. In fact, this slippery slope can go on unchecked for so long that men in their forties have been shown to have morning testosterone levels as low as that of a boy just entering puberty.

ENTERING ANDROPAUSE

Your team is losing, but your coach isn't doing anything about the low T, and your performance keeps getting worse. The medical term for what's happening is a doozy to pronounce, though it's easy to understand once you break it down. It's called hypogonadotropic hypogonadism. *Gonadotropic* refers to your GnRH and LH, your brain hormones. *Gonadism* refers to your testes and, by association, testosterone. *Hypo*, as you know, means low. Luteinizing hormone, gonadotropic releasing hormone, and testosterone all are dropping below what's normal.

Low GnRH + low LH + low testosterone = *hypo*gonadotropic hypogonadism, a downward slide bringing you closer to andropause. This phenomenon typically begins in your late thirties or early forties.

Eventually, testosterone levels drop to such bottom-of-the-barrel lows that the coach has to stop staring at his shoelaces and *do something.* So the hypothalamus and pituitary finally get back in the game. They start producing lots of the brain hormones, GnRH and LH, to compensate. This triggers the production of testosterone. And it works . . . for a little while, anyway. You might get some good runs in; however, your winning streak is likely short-lived. Most of the time your testosterone production gets a little spurt and then falls again.

That's when men enter into andropause. They have a low testosterone and a high LH and GnRH, whereas before they had a low testosterone as well as low LH and GnRH. The medical terminology for andropause is *hyper*gonadotropic hypogonadism.

High GnRH + high LH + low testosterone = andropause. If you are in your fifties, it is likely that you are in andropause or getting close. Don't feel singled out. This shift in hormonal patterns occurs in all men, although the age at which it happens will vary with the individual. I have patients who became andropausal in their late thirties and others who were not yet there in their seventies. A similar hormonal shift is true for women, however, the age range when it occurs is more narrow, from late thirties to late fifties.

You might not notice the effect of andropause each and every day because it starts to feel more like normal life. That's why it's important that you pay attention to your body and the message it's trying to relay. In the next chapter, I'll show you how you can begin to collect more about your personal health history, family history, and lifestyle to optimize your health. By understanding who you are now, you're that much closer to creating a plan to get back to the vitality you felt 20, 30, 40 years ago.

CHAPTER 2

GAME ON! INCREASING HEALTH SPAN

The goal of medicine should be to help you maintain your vitality for life

I n June 2011, Yankees shortstop Derek Jeter, 37, took major heat from New York fans for not playing like he did when he was 27 years old. He couldn't hit the ball as well as he used to. He was striking out too frequently for an elite athlete. He wasn't fast enough to be the brilliant shortstop the fans had come to expect on the field each night. They weren't happy. Neither was Jeter.

The list of legendary athletes who played past their prime is long: Babe Ruth, Joe DiMaggio, Steve Young, Michael Jordan, Shaquille O'Neal, Willie Mays, Mike Tyson, Magic Johnson, Emmitt Smith,

Muhammad Ali, Jerry Rice, and more. It's not easy to find a list of those who decided to call it quits shortly after they reached the peak of their skill level. Swimming champion Michael Phelps is one of the few who comes to mind. Just over a month after his 27th birthday, Phelps swam his final lap on the world stage in the men's 4 x 100-meter Olympic relay. Competing in the butterfly leg of the relay, he went on to win his 22nd gold medal, making him the most decorated Olympian ever. Now Phelps is a self-identified retired Olympic swimmer; in fact, he and his coach Bob Bowman discussed that he wouldn't compete past age 30. (For a while, he was hesitant to even compete in the 2012 summer Olympic Games, after having won eight gold medals in 2008, the most first-place finishes at any one Olympic Game.) What happens next will be up to Phelps, but he has gone on record as saying he will not be competing at the 2016 games in Rio. Phelps knew his superhuman skills were beginning to slip so he had to scale back his participation and the expectations of his fans.

Whether athletes decline more quickly than the rest of us or just appear to because they are so closely watched by owners, coaches, and fans is a big question. Either way, you can learn a lot from how athletes are treated. In 2011, Jeter suffered a calf injury, which put him on the disabled list for the first time since 2003 when he dislocated his shoulder. He received immediate medical attention. All eyes—fans, media, competing teams—were on him. Even without injury, athletes get year-round care. Owners invest millions in trying to keep their athletes in the best shape possible with the top doctors, physical therapists, massage therapists, nutritionists, coaches, exercise physiologists, and trainers. Every avenue is explored to find ways to increase endurance, strength, energy, and acuity in an effort to make all of it last longer than nature might otherwise allow. I thought how great it would be if I could apply that concept, in an integrated fashion, to an aging man or woman in order to make the most of the years they have.

I started exploring this idea further while developing Women's Health at Yale University School of Medicine, realizing I wanted to investigate the world of sports medicine in a setting where being proactive about your health is vital. In 1998, I was asked to lecture at the Aspen Club Sports Medicine Institute, one of the nation's oldest and most respected alternative health care clinics. There, I had a chance to observe firsthand how top athletes are treated by sports medicine clinicians. The experience stuck with me and taught me a great deal. The doctors, along with other specialists, scrutinized over every aspect of the athlete's health, beyond rehabilitation, to optimize his or her performance. It was a prototype that resonated with me, similar to what I had begun at Women's Health, bringing the expertise of a team together proactively. I began to think more about how I could apply this concept to everyone. The truth is, you have great years left—lots of them. Your best years as a small-business owner, doctor, engineer, teacher, lawyer, public servant, parent, or partner may be right now, or perhaps even a decade or more down the line. You want to be sure your mind and body are up to the challenge.

When you think about the course of your life, you've probably wondered about how long you'll live. We all know what a life span is, and we all know it's getting longer with advances in medicine and technology. I focus more on *health span*—the length of time you're living with good quality of life that allows for enjoyment of a long life span. My father's health span lasted up until he died in his nineties. My dad never sat when he could stand, and he never stood still when he could dance. One time, when he was near the end of his life (unbeknownst to him or me), another man asked if he was in his seventies, and seemed to think he was doing great for 70; although he was over 90! When I asked my dad, "Why the dancing and constant moving?" his answer was, "My body feels better if I keep it going actively." It seemed clear to me that this was the way to go.

As a doctor, I feel that my responsibility is to help people dramatically lengthen their health spans, the number of years they enjoy a vibrant, active, youthful, disease-free life. Why have a long life span if you can't live it well? Even to have the drive to stay on your game, you need a basic level of health or you won't be able to push forward and follow a plan to improve the quality of your life. Let's say you have diabetes. You may live to 85 or 90, yet if you don't take care of yourself or improve your carbohydrate metabolism, you may lose your vision or may have to be connected to a dialysis machine. This means having toxins cleared from your body 3 days a week because your kidneys are failing. You're still alive, but how alive? In this case, your health span may run out 25 to 30 years before you die. You don't just want a long life span; you deserve a long health span. The only way to do that is to take a holistic view of your health, and monitoring metabolism and hormones is a critical part of that approach.

In athletes, you see a close-up, high-definition view of your own health span, focused on the time when your body is engineered to be at its physiological best. Because athletes stay within the public eye as they approach middle age, inevitably, as their performance lags, it's easily recognized. It's tough for you to watch; in fact, it feels like a part of you is going down with them. Seeing them in their state of decline makes you aware of your own decline, and that's the last thing you want to notice. You start to ask yourself, *If they look that ridiculous, how must I look?* You let go of Jimmy Connors and embrace Andre Agassi. You let go of Pete Sampras and embrace Rafael Nadal. But wait—in that gap between idols is the moment you could recognize what's happening in your own life. Chances are, though, you blew right past it. You found another dream to cling to, and all was right with the world again. Meanwhile, you can't find another *you,* so instead you turn away from the image in the mirror and cling to the one on your student ID. You're no professional athlete. Still, you'd like to be able to run 5 miles each day, but lately you find yourself winded after 2. You'd like to be able to perform in the bedroom the way you did in your twenties. You might find yourself wondering: *What would it take to get it back?*

CHANGE AND THE IMPORTANCE OF TESTOSTERONE

You are a complicated system made of billions of cells, and those cells communicate with each other. Sometimes, they do so within the same neighborhood, such as within the bone matrix, where cells create and remodel bone. Cells communicate over longer distances, too, from the brain to the testes, for example. The cells in your body are dynamic, adjusting to internal changes, responding to external stimuli, compensating for poor lifestyle choices. This happens as unconsciously and naturally as breathing; it's also completely individual. The combination of experience and genetics is different for each person. You can now actually capture each aspect of your own function, enter the data, and undergo an analysis using the Precision Health Questionnaire (see Appendix).

Let's take a brief step back into high school biology class. Forget Jenny, your crush in the short skirt and Devo T-shirt. Instead, focus on Watson and Crick, the scientists who described the double-stranded structure of the DNA molecule called the double helix. You'll recall that your body's functioning depends upon programming within the double helix. DNA triggers the production of mirror image messenger RNA, which in turn creates specific proteins, hormones, neurotransmitters, or whatever message the RNA is tasked with carrying. You may not be conscious of messages to bump up hormone production or metabolize food in a way that maximizes absorption of nutrients and minimizes oxidative stress. Change in the body occurs very slowly, though it's happening every minute. It's not sudden. There's no huge parting of the seas, no neon sign popping up on the mirror one morning saying, "Your heart attack risk begins now." Transformation happens from nanosecond to nanosecond and accumulates over decades. You're usually not aware of a shift in your health until it all adds up and becomes a visible symptom or disease. It could result in a heart attack at 43 or cancer at 60. Until then, though, your body is adapting all along. You don't pay attention because you take it for granted that your body will continue to do its job.

Sometimes, when you're exposed to something rare, you gain insight with an epiphany about the obvious and everyday. I first became interested in exploring the slowdown in metabolism and hormone production by studying human beings in overdrive, growth happening at warp speed. In 1979 I was conducting research at the National Institutes of Health (NIH) on young boys and girls who were growing up too fast, a condition known as precocious puberty or early adolescence. I was introduced to children who, at age 3 and younger, were having erections and developing biceps. These boys were bigger, stronger, visibly different from their classmates. At age 4 or 5, they had the musculature of a 10-year-old. By the time they reached their 7th or 8th birthday, they looked like teenagers. Parents worried about interactions in the classroom and on the playground. Their sons and daughters were being deprived of their childhoods.

My colleagues and I used GnRH to reverse this biological injustice, giving them time to grow up at a more normal pace. Once we controlled the children's hormone production and put the brakes on this accelerated development, I saw these "adolescents in disguise" turn back into children. It was remarkable. I thought: *We're witnessing maturation and aging in a contracted period of time. We helped these children by altering their production of hormones and slowing their unnaturally rapid development—what if we could prevent or even reverse the process of aging with a similar approach?*

My years of clinical experience since this research on precocious puberty have proven to me that the negative feedback loop—involving the players GnRH, LH, and testosterone—is of critical importance at all stages of life. As you move past your peak reproductive period, usually somewhere between 25 and 30, remember that testosterone production is reduced by 1 to 3 percent each year. The brain *isn't* reacting to those lower T levels by ramping up production of GnRH and LH. Levels of all three hormones are in gradual decline, and this impacts your whole body. Cells in the testes that produce testosterone may be localized; however, they're acting globally. For instance, if you recall, the heart muscle has a significant number of testosterone receptors. If less testosterone is being messengered around the body, there is not enough to bind to the receptors in the organs, like the heart and brain, and perform its intended function. Those receptors become less responsive, or lose receptor binding sites. Without sufficient testosterone levels, you may not regain your strength, and you may be at risk for cardiovascular disease. Your workouts are less effective, and recovery takes longer. But with enough T, I've seen the nearly impossible happen.

Dick DeFluri came into my office when he was 59, shortly after he had a heart attack at 57 that damaged the cardiac muscle. His lab results indicated that he had very low total and free testosterone. For the record, free testosterone is the more clinically meaningful measure, as it denotes the amount of testosterone that's circulating in your body and able to bind to receptor sites. For optimal functioning, free testosterone should fall in the range from 150 to 250 picograms per milliliter (abbreviated pg/mL).

Five years after Dick's heart attack, his cardiologist called me, sounding amazed. It had been 3 years since I helped Dick to optimize his testosterone, getting his free T to more than triple what it was, from 40 to >150 pg/mL. The cardiologist reported that the anterior wall of Dick's heart—the place that had been damaged by the heart attack, as documented by prior tests before starting T—showed no obvious sign of trauma. Conventional wisdom in cardiology is that the damage is visible for the rest of your life. Another measure of cardiac performance is known as the ejection fraction, and it tells me how well your heart is pumping. In Dick's case, his ejection fraction improved as well. Dick's heart recovery was unusual, and while it is anecdotal, I wondered if it was in part due to the increase in Dick's free testosterone, supported by changes in his lifestyle, exercise, and nutrition. Not surprisingly, heart health has improved for many of my patients who have had heart attacks and then began hormone treatment, either with testosterone or human chorionic gonadotropin (hCG). Their cardiologists tell me so. It doesn't always happen this way; yet when I see these findings, I know research assessing such outcomes will follow.

I've cared for so many men with low T that I now know how profound its effect can be. While I can easily spot signs and symptoms, these are often just the tip of the iceberg. As I delve deeper into my patients' backgrounds, family histories, and lifestyles, I discover that many men are at risk for developing disorders of aging like diabetes or osteoporosis. Caught early enough, many of these conditions can be reversed through hormone and metabolic interventions combined with lifestyle changes, supplements, and medications, when clinically indicated. Too often though, I see patients standing at the cliff's edge. At the extreme end of the spectrum are men who are already in free fall; ready or not, they have diabetes or heart disease, though they may be completely unaware. One patient of mine, Larry N. (you'll meet him in the next chapter), had leukemia that went undetected for years. Grappling with illness, the body is not always able to generate hormones at adequate levels. Testosterone is often low with acute and chronic illnesses. Larry's was no exception. At the time of our introduction, he had little to no energy, partly due to the leukemia, certainly, though also likely a result of his testosterone levels being in the basement. While our top priority was getting him to see a specialist, improving his overall health by optimizing his testosterone would only help support his body's ability to respond favorably to treatment for his leukemia.

WHY THERE IS NO SUCH THING AS "NORMAL"

So how do you know where you fall on that spectrum? Are you a Larry N. or a Dick DeFluri? Maybe your situation isn't as dire; still, how can you judge your health right now and ensure a good quality of life going forward?

When doctors judge whether or not you're healthy, they use the parameters established by evidence-based research. Applying that research in a clinical setting, however, often proves challenging. Individual variation is often overlooked. Let's say a medical supply company tests a heart stent for men between 45 and 75 years of age who are experiencing first-time chest pains. The company tells you how many men it tested and tells you how old the men are, but it leaves out one crucial piece of information: The study's investigators have collected a sample of men who are as alike as possible. Why's that? Because each individual is a complex being, and unless the individuals in the study are similar, it is virtually impossible to distinguish the impact of an intervention—there are simply too many variables to control. So researchers of this hypothetical study have aimed to gather a homogeneous group—maybe in addition to being between the ages of 45 and 75, all the men are Caucasian and between 170 and 190 pounds, not too fat or thin.

Now let's say that this stent has a good success rate in the study. What happens when you apply the results of this clinical trial to an entire population? There will be a lot of people for whom the sample won't be representative and so a similar success rate cannot be expected. There can be huge disparities between ethnicities and among men who have different levels of fitness or significantly different diets than those tested. At a cellular level, there will also be variations. Genetics may put certain men at greater or lesser risk of heart disease than those in the study sample. Focusing on the mean misses men who are on either end of what the researchers take to be the normal spectrum. All this means is that applying these findings to every man between the ages of 45 and 75 does not make sense, because outside of the sample population there is great diversity. Even the results of a well-done study published in the *New England Journal of Medicine* will be deficient when it comes to applying them to specific individuals. Yet, it's common practice to retrofit the evidence as best as possible, partly because clinical trials are expensive and there are only so many that can be done. Today, medicine is practiced mostly through a one-size-fits-all filter. All the more reason that it's time for a shift to Precision Medicine, where you, the individual, move into center frame.

There are a few instances where we can *almost* universally apply averages: We know a body temperature above 100 means you're sick, and we know that a hemoglobin A1c level of 6 percent means you're diabetic.

But if you just look at a single screen of your lab results and compare them with somebody else's, you could be falsely reassured. Or, if you're told that your findings are slightly off, it is easy to rationalize the results, attributing them to an off week, a birthday dinner for your son, a celebratory alcohol binge at the office. Remember Livingston Miller? As a trainer, he knew he had to eat every 2 or 3 hours to support high levels of activity. However, his diabetes was obscured by his active lifestyle. Nobody bothered to ask about his family history. Had somebody done so, Livingston's response would have revealed a high incidence of diabetes in most of his first-degree relatives.

THE BELL-SHAPED CURVE AND WHERE YOU FALL

If you look at the testosterone levels in a sample of men at the age of 25, you will see a bell-shaped curve. Some levels are higher, some are lower, and a bunch fall into a larger grouping clustered around the peak. Tests may show that testosterone at 200 pg/mL is right smack in the middle of this spectrum, and it's labeled as an optimal level for any healthy 25-year-old. The problem is that most men don't have their lab results from age 25. Even if they did, circulating and free testosterone are likely not among the biomarkers that would have been ordered. So, if you get your testosterone measured for the first time at age 50 and your doctor says you've fallen nicely into the normal range, what does that mean? Given the fact that the doctor doesn't know your baseline numbers, is the comment useful? No, it is virtually meaningless. Here's why.

If you could look back to discover that you had a testosterone level of 250 pg/mL at your peak as a 25-year-old and it drops to 125 pg/mL at age 50, that is likely to have a significant clinical impact. Compare that to someone who had a testosterone of 150 pg/mL at his peak and it drops down to 100 pg/mL at age 50. Both values are out of the range I like to see, yet the situations differ. If you lose 50 percent of your average free testosterone, this is likely to contribute more to a loss of libido, erectile dysfunction, brain fog, and poor sugar management, along with a massive drop in energy—all changes that are bound to have real implications for your health. Yet if you show up at your doctor's office complaining of symptoms of low T, your doctor is likely going to miss the problem because 125 pg/mL at age 50 looks adequate enough and he or she doesn't know your baseline level. When you rely on the mean while trying to manage the care of the individual, that slice of the bell-shaped curve holds no value. Yet mainstream medicine is often practiced by these guidelines. It's like expecting that every man will fit into a pair of 36-inch pants—not going to happen.

It is important to remember that these averages, however imperfect, are also shifting each decade. That bell-shaped curve may be broad and wide for men in their twenties, and with each decade, as T declines, the curve will skew to the left and may also get narrower and narrower. Even if a doctor tells you, the 50-year-old man with a circulating testosterone of 125, that you're doing just fine, the doctor is comparing you to others within the same age-group. The problem is, we're dealing with aging organisms at failing levels of testosterone. At 50, you're not expected to have a testosterone level of around 200 anymore. But why? In order to optimize your systems, you not only have to remember what you felt like in your twenties and thirties but you also need to consider your biological makeup from those years. By aiming to be "normal" as you age, you're selling yourself short in more ways than one.

What's more, it's fair to assume that if you're being told your testosterone is within range, you're also being told that some of your other lab numbers are normal. I say this because I hear it happen all the time. Here's my question to you: Is being labeled "normal" at every single checkup helping you feel better, other than giving you the false comfort of perhaps thinking, *Okay, I'm not going to die this year*? Probably not. Normal with regard to the mean is likely not normal for you. Good health is more than a series of numbers that are considered acceptable by national guidelines and regulatory bodies.

Now, let's say your numbers are not in the so-called normal range.

You're likely to get some throwaway suggestions that have been repeated so many times they've nearly lost all meaning: "You should exercise a little more." "You really ought to watch what you eat." These recommendations are general and have no regard for who you are, where you live, what your culture is, or what you're doing with your life. For instance, one of my patients, Tony N., exercised nearly every day and was still battling a belly. Telling him to log some extra hours in the gym to keep his weight in check wouldn't have been helpful advice. For Tony, it wasn't the amount of exercise but rather the type that mattered. Tony also had poor eating habits and was not getting enough protein in his diet. As you'll see in subsequent chapters, Tony was a diabetic and had cardiovascular disease, too. Take this example one step further and compare Tony to Livingston. Both worked out, both had diabetes, and both had problems as a result. The symptoms looked very different, however. Tony had a gut and was already in free fall when he met me. As you'll read in Chapter 4, he had a stroke just after our initial phone consultation. Livingston, who was suffering from fainting spells, had a solid physique that belied his silent heart attack. As you'll begin to see, lifestyle, family history, and personal medical history add up in unique ways, creating different symptoms in each individual.

Because you are a complex individual, it follows that your experiences are not one-note. Both Livingston and Tony also had low T, though they led different lives with distinct medical histories. Let's say I asked three men who all had low T (free testosterone hovering around 50) about their perceptions of their sex life. One might say he gets morning erections several times a week, yet he really has no interest in sex and no libido. Another says he has a powerful sex drive, but he can't get it up. The third man may report that his libido is pretty good; he can get it up, but he can't keep it up. If you want to understand testosterone, sexual function, and libido for each of these individual men, there are multiple factors that would feed into these three areas. It's not a one-to-one correlation where if you have low testosterone, you also have no libido, or if you have erectile dysfunction, you never want to engage in sex. The exact same T level in 10 different men will give you 10 different patterns.

YOUR PERSONAL BASELINES
OFFER CRUCIAL HEALTH INSIGHT

While clinical guidelines gathered from research may be of use at a very gross level, there's nothing more effective than monitoring the state of your health by establishing standards that are unique to the functioning of your individual system. How do we do that? By getting your baselines measured as early as possible. Looking at the results of critical tests and tracking variations over time help you to appreciate how you operate. Also, as you'll begin to see, elements of your lifestyle are just as telling as your cholesterol levels or your genetic risk for developing heart disease. It's all important; nothing about your health exists in a vacuum.

It used to be that everyone had a family practitioner who made house calls. The good doctor knew your family history and current health state; frequently he had taken care of you since birth. He might have even taken care of your parents since they were children. That doctor knew your family's history and recognized that different people need distinct kinds of care, both personal and medical. Today, I envision you assembling a team of professionals, the 21st century's equivalent of the family doctor, to help guide you and ensure your well-being. This might involve seeing a primary care physician, a urologist, and a sports medicine specialist. For instance, if you know you're at high risk for developing heart disease, you want to find a cardiologist you trust and establish a relationship with him or her. This way, you're better able to proactively manage your care, perhaps even avoiding an adverse event. If a heart attack or stroke should occur, you know who's going to be treating you. What's more important, that cardiologist (or neurologist or pulmonologist) knows your story, too. There's security in gathering a team of medical professionals whom you trust. They can help you interpret medical data, apply appropriate options, select alternative paths, and ensure that your decisions and choices will work for you. Trust is key, as medical decision making is not a black-and-white science. It is based on judgment and values. The wisdom and knowledge exchanged between you and your team will have a direct impact on the quality of your health throughout your life.

If you think of yourself as a puzzle, you are born with pieces of different shapes and sizes, and those pieces will be arranged just so, depending on your genetic makeup. Your lifestyle changes the way the pieces fit together. In fact, your genes are also dynamic, and decisions you make may have such a profound impact on your health that they actually change the shape of the pieces (more in Chapter 12). The point is that we're all different puzzles, and our pieces can be rearranged and reshaped throughout our lives.

GATHERING YOUR PERSONAL HEALTH METRICS

Putting together the pieces of your puzzle is not unlike assembling a financial portfolio. You wouldn't go into a meeting with your financial advisor without knowing your assets and liabilities, gathering copies of tax returns from the last few years, checking account and credit card statements, insurance policies, and information on your stock holdings and 401(k). My goal is to have you start thinking about your health in the same way.

When you make financial decisions, you consider what you value: buying a less expensive home in the best school district, driving exotic cars instead of going on several vacations, finding a job with a great pension and stock options that will let you retire shortly after 65. These are personal preferences that dictate your financial risk tolerance, which is a well-understood concept. Yet, if you are like most people, your health risk parameters remain a complete unknown. You are satisfied with a rather superficial annual checkup, if that, letting years go by without really assessing your health. One life, lived well, demands attention to the body and mind that house you.

There's a commercial for Prudential Financial Inc., which aired in early 2013. In the ad, people are asked to name the age of the oldest person they know. Then there's some time lapse video as these people put stickers denoting that age on a huge graph. The result: many folks have known someone who has lived into his or her nineties. The ad asks: With the retirement age staying set at 65, how will you be able to afford to live comfortably for the remainder of your life? My question is similar: What will the quality of your life be like in your eighties and nineties? Will your health span keep up with your life span? The answer will depend on how you invest your time, money, and energy in planning for good health in your golden years.

In the financial sector, you have many opportunities for guidance from accountants, investment bankers, stockbrokers, and lawyers. By comparison, Precision Medicine is an expertise with few doctors who practice this level of proactive personalized preventive care. One of the primary functions of this book is to help you assemble a health portfolio that contains as much vital information as your financial portfolio. Let's begin that process with one basic question:

WHO ARE YOU?

You have to answer this before you can start planning for the you that you'd like to be. When I begin the process with a patient, I'm looking at three main areas.

1. MEDICAL HISTORY. What has happened in your past and what is happening right now say a lot about where you're headed and what steps are necessary to optimize your health. There are two directions to explore.

First, we need to help you figure out if you're being treated for the right conditions. Symptoms may look like they're indicating one problem when in reality there may be another underlying issue to blame. What's more, there are connections between different organs in the body that you may not even realize.

For example, you may think a vague ache in your shoulder is innocuous. Your doctor may want to probe further, however, because that ache in your shoulder could mean that something is going on that's affecting your diaphragm. While you remember the backbone being connected to the neck bone, you're pretty sure the deltoid muscle and the diaphragm aren't in direct contact. Yes, that's true; however, the nerves from the

shoulder lead to the diaphragm. If you can't find anything wrong with
the shoulder, your doctor may need to look at the abdomen. You might
have acute pancreatitis causing inflammation, which is irritating your
diaphragm. Then again, it could be what you thought it was: bursitis
caused by a rotator cuff injury you never rehabilitated correctly. Not
only that, you're aggravating it by heavy lifting either at the gym or in
the garden. You may need to see an orthopedist or physical therapist.

Second, you will want to be more conscious about tracking changes
that are occurring in your body, registering the details, and maybe even
jotting down a note or two in your smartphone or on paper. Instead of
brushing off a repetitive sign, you should focus on strengthening your
investigative ability to be aware when it's occurring and how frequently.
Taking notice of these signs and symptoms that alert you to potential
hazards down the road.

For example, blood pressure spikes early in the morning. It's no coin-
cidence that heart attacks happen more commonly then. Around 4:00
or 5:00 a.m., your cortisol—the stress hormone—starts rising in antic-
ipation of getting your body ready to wake up. Your blood pressure goes
up, too. Maybe you're with your new girlfriend, and you're making love
in the morning. Your pulse skyrockets, an artery is partially obstructed,
and suddenly it's too much for your heart; you feel fleeting chest pains.
Later, if you go to your doctor at 1:00 p.m. after you've had a pretty
relaxed morning, and it doesn't bother you to see white coats, your
blood pressure may be fine. That's why it's important to have an understanding of how you feel during different parts of the day. Home in on
the specifics.

Bring your questions and observations to your doctor; however, try to
suggest patterns and be discerning. Maybe every time you eat spicy food,
you have heartburn, or every time you get into an argument at work, you
develop a headache. Perhaps you're getting 8 hours of sleep every night,
yet you're still exhausted. Is it because your work is in turmoil, or your
son didn't get into the college he wanted? Or is it an indication of something less transient? You may have a sleep disorder. Don't write off alterations you feel in your body as no big deal. Be as attuned to minute

observations as you would to the balance in your checking account, and bring up your nagging concerns to your doctor. What's also important is to keep track of your medications as well as vitamins and supplements. Don't rely solely on your doctor (or your partner) to manage this part of your life. Know the pills you're taking, what side effects you've experienced, and how you feel after taking them. You know better than your doctor what it feels like to live in your body.

2. FAMILY HISTORY. Not everybody can undergo a full range of genetic tests, which may be expensive and time consuming. Collecting a family history is the "poor man's" version of a genetic test. In fact, capturing the details of family makeup was a critical component for me when I started treating 40-year-young baby boomers in 1986. I hypothesized that DNA studies would possibly come into play in another 20 years, but my patients couldn't wait that long. So, I thought: *What if I explored their family medical history—diseases, longevity, how their relatives aged, and whatever other details I could muster? What hints would I uncover about their current health and what's awaiting them in the future?* This ended up being a treasure trove of information that helped save lives. It still continues to be useful today even with the leaps and bounds we've made with genetic testing.

Both my parents died fairly young—my mother very young, and my father had medical issues and died shortly thereafter. I lost any family history that was there. I wanted to try to be preventive. One of the elements of Dr. Comite's approach that was attractive to me was that we were going to be looking very deeply. I wasn't just going for a regular checkup where a doctor would say: "Oh, your numbers are okay." With Dr. Comite, we were going to be trying to prevent things from happening, and we would be looking a little bit ahead to see if there were any precursors or warning signs. That was another major key to this.

My wife's dad has been instrumental in my business career. I worked for him for a number of years and he's really been a mentor—well, he's just been diagnosed with Alzheimer's. He is a diabetic, and that he got later in life, so it's kind of put a little bit of a scare into us. This was a guy who took very good care of himself. He's 83, but that's not old today. Especially when 2 years ago he was going up stairs two at a time. So what should I be doing that I'm not doing? It's inevitable that all of us are going to get sick and die. None of us are going to be here forever, but you want to give it the best shot that you possibly can.

—JOHN HORAN, age 57, general contractor

Here's how to start gathering your family history. Ask yourself these questions: What medical issues have your blood relatives dealt with? Does your family have a history of heart disease? Diabetes? Cancer? Look linearly (grandfather, father, you) and laterally (brothers, cousins, and second cousins). With this information, I can fill in the blanks and develop a profile of what medical issues you might inherit that may not have manifested in your day-to-day health. Marathoner Jim Fixx is one of the most famous athletes to die of a sudden heart attack at the age of 52, when the warning signs were right there in his family history. His father had a heart attack at 35 and died of a second one at 43. Fixx's running and high-performance diet likely prolonged his life and gave him a false sense of confidence—he thought he was outsmarting his genetics by doing everything right. Nowadays, a doctor could have obtained genetic tests to find out if he was prone to heart disease. If the findings were positive, he or she could recommend further diagnostic testing and interventions—more fruits and vegetables, interval training with bursts of aerobic activity, aspirin, supplements such as omega-3 fatty acids and CoQ10; medications such as testosterone and a statin—that might have prevented a heart attack. Yet it's very difficult to prevent what you don't know is lurking in the shadows. Records indicate that Fixx hadn't been to see a doctor even though there were early warning signs that he was in trouble. He died way too young as a result.

You can zero in on your genetics by capturing the diagnoses and traits that affect your relatives. You're putting on weight around your trunk, like Uncle Fred, and your mother tells you you're his spitting image. If

Uncle Fred is injecting daily insulin and is on dialysis at 70, diabetes may be lurking in your genes and manifest itself sooner than you might expect, maybe by age 40. You really do want to explore your family's health issues as thoroughly as your own sense of privacy, and that of your relatives, will permit. In the past, relatives may not have been as open about what was wrong as they are now. It was less socially acceptable to speak about illness. It was scary. Perhaps there were superstitions about saying it out loud, as if admitting to the existence of these conditions somehow made them more real. There was a stronger ethos about protecting loved ones from the knowledge of their suffering. Often people would seem to die suddenly when in reality they had been ill for years. Typically, I ask my patients to try to gather a list of the medications prescribed to their immediate family members—parents and grandparents, too, if they're still alive. I understand that it might be more difficult to get your aunts, uncles, and cousins to open their medicine cabinets, but it's worth a try. That information provides incredibly helpful clues.

If you were adopted, your family history may not be available or may be challenging to retrieve. In these cases, genetic assessments might be very useful, given how far they have come. Just make sure you're working with a skilled scientifically based company. There are blood, serum, saliva, and skin tests available. More on this later in Chapters 10 and 12.

3. LIFESTYLE. Twenty-five years ago, I thought that once we had knowledge of genetic makeup we wouldn't require the kind of in-depth metabolic analysis we do for our patients today. I was wrong. Our genetic makeup offers clues; however, it's up to you, with help from this book, to connect the relationships between your genes and the choices you make in work and in play. The pieces do interconnect. Remember the puzzle analogy! Look back at the last year. How do you live? What decisions did you make that directly affected your health in the areas of sleep, stress, sex, diet, and exercise quality? Are you burning the candle at both ends between work and your personal life? What depletes your energy, and what makes you happy? Are you pumping yourself with caffeine during the day and popping a sleeping pill most nights? Are you always up in the air grabbing whatever peanuts the in-flight staff tosses your way, washing them down with a few martinis from the open bar? Are you skipping breakfast? Are you exercising regularly? It may feel like you're filling out a questionnaire for a psychologist, but remember, your state of mind and everyday habits directly impact the production of hormones and the function of your organs.

You have no control over your father's prostate cancer or your mother's heart disease. You do have control over the food you put in your mouth and whether or not you drink or smoke. This is a critically important concept for all of us. Lifestyle factors are now being shown to directly affect changes in the way our genes perform and produce proteins. It is not just another far-fetched hypothesis; data is accumulating that suggests this is so. To optimize your health, you have to begin where you are by understanding your behaviors and how you actually live—*as opposed to how you think you live.* You may think you're making healthy decisions, when in reality you're not. You may think you're dealing effectively with stress, yet your body might not be adapting quite as well as you believe. I have found this kind of gap in understanding in every kind of man, from a man who does little to sustain his health to the most ambitious athlete.

What is your own sense of your health at this point? What bothers you the most at this time of your life? Here are some of the concerns I have heard, derived from my experience treating men over the last couple of decades.

• Metabolism that doesn't work like it used to, making weight loss difficult

• Lack of energy

• Lost sense of invulnerability and certainty

• Few morning erections

• Inability to get and/or sustain an erection

• Diminished libido, with sex no longer being a top priority

- Lack of sharpness in thinking

- Joint weakness

- Too many aches and pains

- Knees and back that hurt most of the time

- Reduced stamina and endurance for exercise

- Too long a recovery after exercising

- Slow recovery from injury

- No interest in going to parties, a night out on the town, or partaking in activities outside of work

How many of these problems sound familiar? Perhaps you're just now noticing that one or more have been bothering you for years. Any one of these reduces your potential health span, though its effects are likely reversible. Recovering function in multiple aspects of life is possible; my patients report so every day. This is what drives me to do the work I do.

READY FOR ACTION

In my practice, before I ever see or speak to a patient for the first time, I review a lengthy, detailed Precision Health Questionnaire (PHQ) that he has already filled out. This document has evolved over many years from my clinical experience and medical necessity. Each section asks you something about yourself that you and your doctor need to know about your current and future health.

For the book, I've created a somewhat condensed version of the PHQ that you can use. The next thing you're going to do is collect data—your personal health metrics—by filling in the PHQ (which can be found in the Appendix). You might look at these questions and think, *I fill out this kind of form for every doctor I see, and then nobody refers to it ever again*. Not this time, because your personal metrics will become as crucial to the equation of maximizing your health span as your lab results.

From your answers, you'll have a better understanding of how to partner with your doctor to interpret the next steps you need to take. You will be able to use the data you collect. You can even upload it onto the Web site KeepItUpTheBook.com. These can then be turned into next steps with your personal doctor, if indicated. Instead of putting you on a one-size-fits-all program, I am going to provide parameters, particular for you, that will act as guidelines to achieving optimal health.

Think about how you can mobilize yourself by filing out this questionnaire to reach your goals. Refer to the Appendix for the PHQ, or, alternatively, you may go to KeepItUpTheBook.com.

CHAPTER 3

THE METABOLIC TESTS

Find out how well or poorly your body's engine is humming

I had just turned 50. As a triathlete and a reporter who covers sports and fitness, I figured I was doing everything right health-wise and was much fitter than most guys my age. I exercised regularly, had annual checkups, and because of my career I knew more about health and nutrition than the average man. So you can imagine my shock when I got the results of pretty extensive blood work. I was prediabetic and wouldn't have known it if I didn't have a hemoglobin A1c blood test. That was a wake-up call. Further testing showed that I carried a gene defect for a rare heart condition. Without this knowledge, I would have thought I was in perfect health.

—JIM C., age 51, writer

Tom Brokaw broke the news to the nation: Tim Russert, the famous broadcaster who moderated *Meet the Press* for more 16 years, had collapsed and died of a sudden heart attack on the floor of the WRC-TV radio offices. Doctors reported that Russert's recent stress test had shown no cause for alarm, and that he had begun exercising to lose weight. What if his doctors had explored deeper, beyond the obvious belly fat and battery of tests? Russert's story may stand out, but it doesn't stand alone. There are plenty of men who die unexpectedly at a young age, even those who differ from Tim Russert. I remember watching Tim as I ran on the treadmill Sundays, wondering whether he even knew the risks he faced being clearly out of shape with a demanding career. Yet many more men, just like Jim C., exercise regularly, look great, eat well, even run marathons, yet die suddenly just like Tim.

As a young doctor doing research, I would talk with potential study participants and get to know them before ordering tests. I would ask many questions that might have been intrusive; however, I was young, so I didn't know better. But my naïveté paid off. The more I knew about each patient, the more specific I could be in assessing him. Years later, these same patients would often come back to me because their bodies and minds were not functioning like they used to. They felt anxieties they never had earlier; they were putting on weight and didn't know why; they felt like they couldn't keep up with all their obligations at the office or at home; and they couldn't find any reason for these vicissitudes. By just looking at their previous lab results, I couldn't figure it out either. I needed to know more.

It prompted me to step back and say, "I can't answer your questions because I don't know enough about you." Doctors generally don't like to admit that we don't have solutions. Yet, it's often true. We often don't know enough just from lab results measured against reported norms. Remember, each individual is a unique puzzle. I have my patients help me collect the relevant data that tell me who they were and who they are, based on personal medical history, family history, and lifestyle. This allows me to create a context to better understand their particular stats, reverse potential risks, and take them to the next level. Even so, I won't have all the answers. I don't know what I don't know. Still, I am better able to advise when I understand the background, goals, and feelings of the person I'm treating. I want to deliver on the same kind of care I give to my own family and loved ones, as if my patient is my father or son. I begin with metabolism because it is so pervasive; if yours is not functioning properly, your health foundation is undermined. Most doctors explore metabolism through blood work, although it's typically limited in scope.

With labs I order for patients, I focus on several aspects of systemic function—including sugar metabolism and kidney and liver biomarkers, cholesterol, complete blood counts, inflammatory markers, and hormones. When you combine the results with the patient's lifestyle, history, and symptoms, it lays the groundwork for the path to optimizing health. It may also give clues to indicate a disease that is brewing or already evident.

For instance, let's say I discovered that your uric acid is borderline elevated at 8.0 milligrams per deciliter (mg/dL). Then when I ask you about your diet, you report that you're eating shellfish several times a week and having a glass or two of red wine daily. You also tell me that your father had gout. All signs would suggest that you might be on your way to having a gouty arthritis attack in the future. On the other hand, your blood work may serve as a kind of system of checks and balances, giving us insight that may refute evidence in your family history, genetics, and lifestyle. For instance, your mother may be diabetic, your father died of a heart attack, and yet your blood sugar and cholesterol are in an ideal range. This is great news. Of course, given your history, we would want to make sure your cholesterol levels stay that way by monitoring your health over time. Or we would check that other markers, which may be harder to detect, are not awry (more on that in Chapter 10).

Within metabolism, I look at these specific areas, among others:

Carbohydrates

Liver and kidney function

Lipids profile

Complete blood count (CBC) (see page 58)

Inflammatory markers

Bone studies

Below, I will explain the tests that help me evaluate each area.

CARBOHYDRATE METABOLISM
TESTS: FASTING BLOOD SUGAR, FASTING INSULIN, HEMOGLOBIN A1C

Your body uses carbohydrates as energy. However, if you load up on starchy foods—bread, pasta, cereal, pretzels, crackers, potato chips—as well as cakes or candy, you store all that energy as fat and may run into a host of medical problems, including diabetes.

Adult-onset diabetes is on the rise, afflicting 26 million individuals in the United States. That figure has shot up exponentially over the past 30 years. Predictions indicate that one in three adults in the United States will have diabetes by 2050. These odds roughly suggest that either you or one of your two best friends will be a diabetic. Not good. The projected cost is more than $500 billion spent on treatment alone by 2020. That doesn't include the cost of all the disabilities that result from diabetes nor the burden (financial, personal, and emotional) on the individual and his family.

Most doctors use a single blood test to look for diabetes or prediabetes (fasting glucose). In my practice, I include a fasting insulin test as well.

The thinking around carbohydrate metabolism has changed. Twenty-five years ago, you could have a fasting blood sugar level as high as 110 mg/dL and be considered only borderline high. Now we know that fasting blood sugar should be in the 80s with an upper limit of 95 mg/dL. In fact, I aim to have my patients with levels that fall between 70 and 80 mg/dL. Insulin is released into the blood to metabolize sugar from food and should be undetectable after a 12-hour fast. With no food in the system, no insulin should be produced. If it's present, that indicates insulin resistance.

I like to see the relationship between sets of numbers. These tests show a very narrow slice of your carbohydrate metabolism and can be skewed by how you ate and exercised the day before. Eat a big plate of penne vodka (pure carbs, complex sugar) paired with several glasses of red wine (pure sugar), and you'll have elevated readings in the morning. A meal of lean meat and steamed vegetables the night before, however, might yield lower numbers that fall in a more acceptable range.

What is more helpful is measuring fasting blood sugar and fasting insulin in addition to a biomarker that shows how you metabolize sugar over time. This is known as hemoglobin A1c, which the American Diabetes Association began using routinely only in 2010 to diagnose diabetes. Often, as with Jim C., it was only by adding hemoglobin A1c that I was able to detect a patient's prediabetic condition. Hemoglobin A1c tells us how the body metabolizes carbs over a 3-month period. I integrate this information with facts about the patient's diet, exercise, genetics, and hormones such as testosterone, insulin, and cortisol.

Hemoglobin A1c reflects the state of your sugar metabolism by assessing the stickiness of your red blood cells (RBCs). Red blood cells live for approximately 100 days, and sugar adheres to those cells. Picture a red blood cell with sugar on it. The more sprinkles you have stuck to your RBCs, the more the cells look like sugarcoated jelly doughnuts. If your body is having a hard time clearing sugar from your blood, your hemoglobin A1c level will be high. The higher your score, the greater your risk of diabetes. National guidelines for hemoglobin A1c have recently been lowered. Now a score of 6 percent is considered an indication of diabetes, while 5.7 denotes prediabetes. A score of 5 percent or lower is ideal for both longevity and health.

It is common for individuals to be first told by their doctor they are diabetic when their blood sugar is well over 150 mg/dL, and by that time their hemoglobin A1c measure may be 7.5 percent or higher. Typically, there are no visible signs of diabetes, although some people report feeling thirstier or needing to urinate more often. Many times, an acute infection will unmask diabetes. In part, this is because people with diabetes don't respond as well to infections and end up far sicker than those without the disorder.

Many men are told to "just watch" their blood sugar, though their doctor may admit their levels are "a little high." Consequently, nothing is done to intervene.

Stanley W.,
AGE 45, COLLEGE PROFESSOR

Chief medical concerns: diabetes

Family history: diabetes, cardiovascular disease, high blood pressure

Lifestyle: too many drinks; regular workouts, albeit unproductive; too many carbs; depression; problems with sexual function

Goals: lose weight, improve sexual function, regain stamina

Stanley W. is an academician who has taught calculus at a local university for 2 decades. He was recently diagnosed with diabetes, though he was trying to manage it by making lifestyle adjustments. Stan lives with his wife, Madeline, who is a sommelier. They have two older children—a daughter and a son. Cardiovascular disease, diabetes, and high blood pressure all run in his family.

At 45, Stan loved sharing a bottle of wine most nights over dinner with his wife, and he wasn't particularly concerned with what he was eating. He regularly ate pasta and had a sweet tooth. Recently, he started training with our exercise physiologist, Steven Villagomez, and was excited about getting back into shape and losing weight. Stan was frustrated that he couldn't put on lean muscle despite his twice-a-week regimen of resistance training mixed with interval training. Interval training is particularly good for people with diabetes because it preserves muscle and burns carbs. With Stan's overindulgent lifestyle, getting into shape was a losing battle. In addition to his frustration at the gym, Stan also suffered from depression, low libido, and erectile dysfunction.

Our exercise physiologist, Steven, suspected that Stan's case wasn't being handled as aggressively as possible, even though he also knew that

Stan wasn't doing all that he was supposed to. He asked to see Stan's lab results from his endocrinologist, and then recommended that Stan come to the office for a thorough health analysis, particularly because Stan was young, yet not going in the right direction. Stan's glucose metabolism was poor, and—combined with his lifestyle and a finding of low testosterone— it was clear that Stan needed to make some changes. His fasting glucose was 146 mg/dL, fasting insulin was at 7 mcIU/mL, and hemoglobin A1c was at 7.7 percent—all too high. His urinalysis also revealed protein in his urine, which is associated with diabetes. While we helped Stan improve his diabetes, his goals included losing weight, improving his sexual function, and being able to work out without exhaustion. Here are Stan's numbers.

Chemistry Screen (focus on carbohydrate metabolism)

TEST	LOW	HIGH	STAN'S NUMBERS
Glucose	65	95	146↑*
Hemoglobin A1c	3.5	5.1	7.7↑*
Insulin	1	5	7↑*

* = abnormal, out of range

KIDNEY AND LIVER BIOMARKERS

TESTS: URINALYSIS, URIC ACID, ASPARTATE AMINOTRANSFERASE (AST), ALANINE TRANSAMINASE (ALT), GAMMA-GLUTAMYL TRANSPEPTIDASE (GGTP)

Every day your body performs many functions to maintain balance, or homeostasis. It automatically adjusts temperature to the environment or to illness, mobilizes the production of proteins and sugar to burn as fuel, stores carbohydrates as fat for use during lean times, and oxygenates your blood.

One of the most important functions that the body engages in to maintain homeostasis is clearing toxins—breaking down the waste from food, medications, supplements, and everything else we consume. This is the job of the liver and kidneys. The tests listed above will tell your doctor how well your organs are functioning. A low or high result will prompt your doctor to explore possible causes, which may include gallstones, viruses, or too much alcohol, diet, or disease.

URINALYSIS. A urinalysis examines the elements of your urine. As your kidneys clear protein, calcium, and glucose. Problems may occur that may result in traces of blood in the urine. The test may indicate whether there is a risk of cancer or stones, or if an infection is present.

PATIENT PROFILE

Robert R.,
AGE 46, PSYCHOLOGIST

Chief medical concerns: kidney stones

Family history: cancer

Lifestyle: depression, little exercise after spinal surgery, strict diet, mild sleep apnea, issues with sexual function

Goals: exercise regularly, lose weight, recapture libido and sexual function

Despite having a strong support network of family and friends as well as an exciting new career venture, Robert R.'s quality of life had been diminishing for nearly a decade. Things came to a head once he made a midlife career switch and decided to become a therapist after years of working in television media. It was tough to keep up in graduate school at 46, when most of his classmates were nearly 20 years younger. Robert also recently underwent surgery on his spine, which brought further stress into his life and prevented him from exercising, something he had previously enjoyed. Lately, he was growing despondent.

Even prior to the operation, Robert had his share of health issues including weight gain, mild sleep apnea, problems with sexual function, and bouts of gout. Most troubling of all, cancer ran deep in his family history, touching his brother and claiming the lives of his mother and father.

When Robert came in to see me in the fall of 2011, he mentioned having a history of passing a kidney stone. This admission was confirmed by the results of his urinalysis, which showed traces of blood in his urine. When I see this, the most serious possibility is cancer in the genitourinary tract—most commonly from the kidneys to the bladder. Given his family's history of cancer and Robert's deteriorating health, I wanted to rule out this diagnosis. Another possibility was that the blood in his urine (known as hematuria) was induced by sexual intercourse in the prior 72 hours, or by the presence of a stone, which irritates the interior of the kidney.

Robert was focused on improving his quality of life overall. But first we had to tackle his kidney stones. Indeed, I determined that Robert has kidney stones, as his lab test revealed an elevated uric acid level of 9 mg/dL. A repeat urinalysis was requested, and no evidence of blood was found. Robert had abstained from sexual intercourse for 3 days. With better metabolic function, he would have more energy to increase his exercise, which would also have a positive impact on depression, desire, and sexual function.

Urinalysis

TEST	LOW	HIGH	ROBERT'S NUMBERS
Color	N/A	N/A	Yellow
Appearance	N/A	N/A	Clear
Specific Gravity	1.001	1.035	1.015
Protein	0	Trace	Negative
Glucose	0	5	Negative
Ketones	0	0	Negative
Blood	0	0	**Small***
Bilirubin	0	0	Negative
Nitrites	0	0	Negative
Leukocytes	0	0	Negative
WBC	0	5	0
Epithelial Cells	0	20	None
RBC	0	5	0–1
Bacteria	0	0	Few

* = abnormal, out of range

URIC ACID. Gout is a common problem that arises when the kidneys have trouble clearing toxins. Uric acid deposits may develop in your body, the most common sites being the joints of the big toes, elbows, and knees. Gouty arthritis often is excruciatingly painful and is linked to drinking too much red wine, as you'll see in Rajiv S.'s story below. It may be related to eating too much cheese, shellfish, or spinach. There's a genetic predisposition, too, yet typically diet is the key trigger to an attack, which will manifest in intense arthritic pain or kidney stones. If you know that someone in your family has had a gout attack, and your uric acid levels are on the higher end of the spectrum, it might be best to switch from spinach to arugula and cut back on the red wine, even if you are in Italy.

PATIENT PROFILE

Rajiv S.,
AGE 59, CFO

Chief medical concerns: gout and diabetes

Family history: gout, arthritis, heart attack, diabetes

Lifestyle: infrequent exercise, cigarettes (two packs/week), too much red wine

Goals: regain energy, manage diabetes, look and feel younger

Rajiv S. was approaching 60 and had done his research on antiaging. He realized that superficial changes, like those produced by Botox or facelifts, were easier than correcting what was wrong with aspects you can't scrutinize in a mirror. Still, he felt like, in general, society viewed aging as a disease, and he wanted to do something to fix it, something that went beyond the purview of a plastic surgeon or dermatologist.

A successful CFO, Rajiv said he didn't regularly schedule time for exercising. When he got a free moment, he enjoyed hiking and taking yoga classes. He was struggling with a high cholesterol and poor carbohydrate metabolism and was skeptical about taking prescription medications.

His habits were catching up with him as well. Rajiv had smoked two packs of cigarettes per week for the past 30 years. He also frequently drank red wine, which he believed to be beneficial. The problem wasn't so much his choice of beverage as the quantity. Having two or three glasses a few times a week meant that the risk of the sugar outweighed the benefit of the antioxidant. His alcohol consumption was contributing to his gout and diabetes.

Rajiv had gotten an earlier blood draw that revealed that his fasting glucose was 101 mg/dL. "Only 101!" he said when he came into my office, "That's not bad." However, my team and I explained to him, as I've explained to you, that the guidelines have shifted. Now anything at 95 mg/dL or higher is considered diabetic. Also, his hemoglobin A1c was at 6.1 percent, which also confirmed a diagnosis of diabetes. His fasting insulin was at 7 mcIU/mL, further indicating insulin resistance. Even though he denied having any overt symptoms of gout, his uric acid levels were very high, and, when prompted, he recalled past attacks affecting his big toes. Also, when we asked about his family history, he reported that his mother had a 10-year history with gout and arthritis. Cardiovascular disease was another concern. His father, who had "borderline" diabetes, died early of a heart attack, and his sister had one at 50. I needed to bring down his cholesterol levels. Underpinning all of these issues, his low hormone levels were typical of hypogonadatropic hypogonadism (low T, LH, and GnRH) and growth hormone (GH) deficiency.

Rajiv's goal was straightforward: He wanted to reverse the disorders of aging and regain his energy levels. Moreover, he was worried about living with diabetes.

Chemistry Screen

TEST	LOW	HIGH	RAJIV'S NUMBERS
Glucose	65	95	**101↑***
Hemoglobin A1c	3.5	5.1	**6.1↑***
Insulin	1	5	**7↑***
Blood Urea Nitrogen (BUN)	7	25	16
Creatinine (Cr, serum)	0.5	1.4	0.93
Uric Acid	1.7	8.2	**8.3↑***

* = abnormal, out of range

AST, ALT, AND GGTP. The liver sits just underneath your diaphragm on your right side. Its main job is to sift through whatever you've ingested—food, drink, supplements, medications—and distribute the good stuff through the blood while sending the bad stuff on its way to being disposed of as waste. The liver is also the main site for glucose exchange, or converting sugar into energy. It manages the storage of glucose in muscle and the creation of fat to handle excess sugar.

Liver function tests, including AST, ALT, and GGTP, tell us if you've had viruses like hepatitis, Epstein-Barr, and mononucleosis, or if you've got fatty deposits that tax the liver's ability to clear toxins efficiently. These tests also can show if you're drinking too much alcohol. Overconsumption can lead to abnormal liver function and ultimately cirrhosis, a condition that scars the organ and severely impairs its function. Elevated liver biomarker levels may suggest that you're not processing medications well, or a bump in the numbers may be transient, signifying that you're struggling with a common cold.

You may already know that when the whites of your eyes are yellow, your stool is white, and your urine is dark, you're clearing bilirubin, a product of the breakdown of toxins from your liver. There's a backup of what your liver and gallbladder can handle, and bilirubin spills into your blood, turning everything the wrong color. If you're iron deficient, it can be another sign of liver trouble. Iron overload, or hemochromatosis, will also interfere with liver function.

There are hereditary conditions that can lead to cirrhosis; still, overconsumption of alcohol and hepatitis usually lead the list. There are various forms of hepatitis; certain kinds you get from shellfish while others are transmitted through bodily fluids, anything from blood transfusions and needles to sexual activity. Hepatitis may also lie dormant for years, as you'll see in Phillip B.'s story on the following page, and may manifest in liver disease.

PATIENT PROFILE

Phillip B.,
AGE 58, INTERNATIONAL SALES MANAGER

Chief medical concerns: hepatitis C, overweight

Family history: liver cirrhosis, substance abuse

Lifestyle: no exercise ever since knee injury; poor diet; too much alcohol

Goals: manage hepatitis C, maintain energy to keep up with jet-setting lifestyle, lose weight

At 58, Phillip B. was living out his life on different coasts. In the 1980s, he had headed up a project with a successful international company in Atlanta, GA, where he met and married his wife. When their children became teenagers, Phillip chose to move his family to a suburb about 45 minutes outside Seattle, where he had spent his "wonder years."

During this transition in 2008, Phillip was stressed, not eating right, and not exercising, the last of which was partly due to a prior knee injury a few years earlier. He was 30 pounds overweight and recently noticed that he had to urinate frequently, signifying he might have diabetes. Drinking—whether at a business dinner or in the airport on a layover—was a constant in Phillip's life. He often drank five glasses of wine in a single sitting at least a couple of times a week. For him, this was cutting back. What's more, Philip's family had a history of substance abuse, and he had a grandfather who died of cirrhosis, the result of heavy drinking.

When Phillip came to my office, he was somewhat overweight, yet his major complaint was a lack of energy, and lately, several bouts of vertigo and ringing in his ears. In addition to high cholesterol and poor carb metabolism, his lab results had shown elevated AST, ALT, and GGTP—all biomarkers of liver function. And they weren't just a little out of range, they were quite elevated.

I've seen it happen where a patient looks relatively healthy and claims to be asymptomatic, yet his labs reveal an underlying problem. Everything

(continued)

begins to align once we add in family history, personal history, and notes about lifestyle. Sometimes there's a piece of information the patient is reluctant to share, despite its critical importance to his health. In other cases, he just doesn't think to mention it because it happened so long ago. This was the case with Phillip. The choices he made more than 25 years ago were actually affecting him today. In college Phillip had used recreational drugs, including cocaine via injection. While the drinking continued into middle age, he said he had stopped using drugs in his twenties. It wasn't until after his diagnosis, when he was calling one of his closest college buddies, that he found out that another had died as a result of hepatitis C. Phillip likely had the virus as well as all his friends who had shared supplies in college.

A diagnosis of hep C would explain why his vestibular system was thrown off. It also made sense that his liver biomarkers were all high; they had likely been inching upward for some time, the result of Phillip going years without detection of hep C.

Phillip came in looking to maximize his health now that he was moving back and forth between cities; he wanted to lose weight. Our primary goal to start, however, was to manage the disease that was attacking his liver. By treating the virus, his baseline numbers improved, as seen below.

Chemistry Screen

TEST	LOW	HIGH	PHILLIP'S NUMBERS
Glucose	65	95	73
Hemoglobin A1c	3.5	5.1	6.7♠*
Insulin	1	5	14♠*
Bilirubin, Total	0.2	1.5	0.6
Bilirubin, Direct	0	0.3	0.2
Alkaline Phosphatase	20	125	73
GGTP	3	80	151♠*
Lactate Dehydrogenase (LD)	100	250	179
AST (SGOT) u/l	3	50	124♠*
ALT (SGPT)	3	60	206♠*

* = abnormal, out of range

FATTY LIVER DISEASE. Fatty liver is in condition in which the liver is damaged in some way and, instead of having active cells, deposits of fat develop and impair function. Alcohol could be the underlying cause, as could diabetes. Fatty liver deposits can be detected with an ultrasound. If you have them, you likely have a problem with your carbohydrate metabolism and will need medication to manage your glucose and insulin. You'll also need to implement some lifestyle changes. Of note, it's believed that nonalcoholic fatty liver disease (NAFLD) is the most prevalent liver disorder in the United States, and it's linked to insulin resistance. It's called *nonalcoholic* because most people that have it do not abuse alcohol, and so liver damage isn't alcohol related. You may not realize you have NAFLD, as most people don't experience any tenderness or pain.

PATIENT PROFILE

Jensen D.,
AGE 50, AUTOMOTIVE SALESMAN

Chief medical concerns: fatty liver infiltrates, concomitant to diabetes

Family history: high blood pressure, cancer, heart attack, hormone imbalances

Lifestyle: diet full of junk food, high stress, little sleep, no exercise, marital problems

Goals: lose weight, create an regular exercise program

When the economy crashed in September 2008, Jensen D. was living in a Detroit suburb and working for the automotive industry. His pressure increased tenfold as the city was turning into an industrial ghost town. His diet was poor and he stopped going to the gym. At home, his wife claimed Jensen wasn't spending enough time with the kids and made him shuttle his two young girls to soccer and karate, often picking up McDonald's along the way. At night, after he read bedtime stories to his girls, the TV would be his only companion.

(continued)

Jensen's family history was full of worrisome concerns: cancer, heart attacks, high blood pressure, and hormone imbalances. In fact, when Jensen came into the office, he had a positive review of symptoms. Essentially that means that everything hurt. He was sensitive to light, especially the spots on the showroom floors and the fluorescents overhead. He had tingling in his left arm, issues with sexual function, and heart palpitations during his morning commute.

Jensen's labs showed low testosterone, no doubt contributing to his low libido. His free testosterone was at 50 picograms per milliliter (pg/mL), which is equivalent to that of the testosterone levels of a boy in puberty. His blood work also indicated that he had diabetes, with high cholesterol and hypertension as well. Most important, however, his blood work showed that he had an elevated ALT. His was 74 IU/L; we like to see folks under 55 IU/L. This number signified that Jensen already had fatty deposits on his liver, which was likely attributable to his diabetes and could lead to cirrhosis. (An ultrasound test of Jensen's liver confirmed that diagnosis.)

Once he found out his carbohydrate and cholesterol profile were out of range, Jensen's goals were to get back into shape, improve his diet, and lose weight. He wanted to design an exercise program that would help him build lean muscle.

Chemistry Screen

TEST	LOW	HIGH	JENSEN'S NUMBERS
Glucose	65	95	91
Hemoglobin A1c	3.5	5.1	**6.7↑***
Insulin	1	5	5
Uric Acid	1.7	8.2	4.9
Bilirubin, Total	0.2	1.5	0.7
Bilirubin, Direct	0	0.3	0.1
Alkaline Phosphatase	20	125	62
GGTP	3	80	53
Lactate Dehydrogenase (LD)	100	250	242
AST (SGOT) u/l	3	50	35
ALT (SGPT)	3	60	**74↑***

* = abnormal, out of range

LIPIDS

TESTS: TOTAL CHOLESTEROL, HDL AND LDL, TRIGLYCERIDES, CORONARY RISK RATIO

The practice of medicine changes about every 10 years as we learn new facts through experience and research. At one time, it was acceptable to have a total cholesterol level of 250 mg/dL. Certainly that number wasn't ideal. Now guidelines are a little stricter, so that 200 mg/dL or lower is the goal for most folks who are not at risk. I like patients to aim for a total cholesterol of 140 to 170 mg/dL. I also like for men to know their HDL and LDL—which are components of the total cholesterol—even though those stats are just the tip of the iceberg (as you will see in Chapter 10).

The reason you want higher good HDL cholesterol is that it blocks whatever damage the bad LDL cholesterol might do. HDL is also a positive indicator of longevity. You'll want to aim to have an HDL greater than 50 mg/dL, though the higher the better. As with total cholesterol levels, the mainstream medical community used to think that an LDL of 130 mg/dL was acceptable. Now we know better. Disease occurs more frequently with an LDL of 130, and you may be at risk for a heart attack. National guidelines recommend that your LDL stay under 100. Multiple risk factors modify those recommendations. I urge my patients to keep their LDL around 70 and encourage them to get that number down to 40 if they have other significant risk factors, like prediabetes, high blood pressure, and/or a family member who has cardiovascular disease.

Estimates from the Centers for Disease Control and Prevention (CDC) from 2010 show that 16 percent of the US adult population has high cholesterol, and 37 percent (or 81.1 million Americans) has cardiovascular disease. While cholesterol can be an indicator of heart disease, as with all biomarkers, you have to look at this measure in relation to lifestyle, personal history, and family history, as well as new research that keeps refining what we know. If you have additional risk factors, then digging deeper is essential.

TRIGLYCERIDES. Triglycerides are another type of fat in the bloodstream that has to be taken into account when looking at cholesterol—especially if you have a family history of heart disease. Elevated triglycerides have little to do with how much fat or dietary cholesterol you consume and more to do with your sugar intake and your activity levels. A high triglyceride score—greater than 100 mg/dL, and definitely, 150 mg/dL—should have you examine blood sugar, insulin, and how your body metabolizes glucose. Triglycerides can also impact the results of your cholesterol panel, making it difficult to read. Such was the case with Dave M.

PATIENT PROFILE

Dave M.,
AGE 48, HOSPITAL COO

Chief medical concerns: high cholesterol, obesity

Family history: cardiovascular disease, stroke, diabetes, arthritis

Lifestyle: fluctuations in weight; weight gain; stress derived from dealing with his father's illnesses

Goals: compete in a triathlon

A lacrosse player in high school; a football star in college; and a marathon competitor in business school, Dave M. grew up active and stayed that way. Lately though, Dave had been feeling his 48 years, and he was struggling to care for his father, who had a host of medical issues including cardiovascular disease, diabetes, rheumatoid arthritis, and was also recovering from a stroke. Dave had relocated to Maine to care for him. His father wasn't good at fending for himself, as Dave's mother had unexpectedly passed away with a sudden heart attack a year prior.

At the same time, Dave was struggling to keep off weight. He had tried various diets—one where he consumed only 600 calories a day, another consisting only of juice and protein shakes. Despite his efforts, Dave had put on an additional 25 pounds while he was managing his father's care remotely and traveling back and forth across state lines, stopping frequently at rest stops and getting fast food in addition to coffee. A recent knee injury made exercising difficult.

Watching what his father went through, Dave grew jaded by the medical system and its red tape. He didn't trust doctors and didn't want to be around them, yet he also knew he needed help. When he came into my office in 2010, he was teetering on obesity. He knew his high cholesterol levels were a significant contributing factor to his risk of stroke and heart attack, particularly in light of his parent's medical conditions. He was right.

His blood work prior to his visit revealed several potential concerns, specifically with his lipids, cholesterol as well as triglycerides. He had what's known as a dyslipidemic profile, which means that there's more than one measure that's out of range.

Doctors routinely look at your total cholesterol and triglycerides, often your HDL and LDL, too. The bad cholesterol, LDL, isn't actually measured in your blood; it's typically calculated. And if your triglycerides are too high (usually greater than 400 mg/dL), then you can't calculate your LDL. This was the case with Dave. Additionally, his HDL was too low, at 28 mg/dL. That is why I ordered some additional tests to get the full picture. In addition to his testosterone, other hormones, such as dihydrotestosterone and DHEA, were also at less than acceptable levels. (More on those in Chapter 4.)

Dave's new goal is to compete in a triathlon, and he hoped that being on the program would give him the energy to push himself during training.

Lipid Panel

TEST	LOW	HIGH	DAVE'S NUMBERS
Non-HDL Cholesterol	0	100	128
Cholesterol	0	200	156
Triglycerides	0	100	438↑*
HDL	50	200	28↓*
LDL, calculated	0	100	N/A†
Coronary Risk Ratio	1	3.5	5.57↑*
Cholesterol, VLDL	4	40	NA†

* = abnormal, out of range

†Because Dave's triglycerides were so high, his LDL and VLDL could not be calculated.

COMPLETE BLOOD COUNT
TEST: CBC

If you're a fan of medical dramas, I'm sure you've heard the term "CBC" thrown around. It stands for complete blood count, and it measures the number of cells in a given blood sample. On a global level, it looks at white blood cells (WBCs) and red blood cells (RBCs), though there are almost 20 different markers that allow me to interpret what might be going on in your immune system.

An elevated or decreased WBC count can be indicative of simple infections like sinusitis or diseases like cancer and HIV-AIDS. I can also see what kind of infection you have by looking at neutrophils and lymphocytes, which are part of a CBC. If neutrophils are high and lymphocytes are low, you could have a bacterial infection. If neutrophils are low and lymphocytes are high, this could signal viral infection. As you'll see in the following story, Larry N.'s lymphocytes were so high that they signaled something beyond a virus.

PATIENT PROFILE

Larry N.,
AGE 61, ENGINEER

Chief medical concerns: leukemia

Family history: leukemia, Down syndrome

Lifestyle: poor diet, little exercise, frequent traveling

Goals: refer to hematologist, strengthen immune system, raise energy levels

At 61, Larry N. was a grandparent three times over, and he spent his days managing his own engineering firm—its specialty was roller coaster design for amusement parks. He had his bad habits—not eating right, not working out—and his life was stressful. He made frequent trips around the nation to meet with contractors and test-ride the coasters (a definite perk of the job).

Larry's parents had been in excellent health, both living into their nineties. His siblings, however, weren't so lucky. His sister was diagnosed with chronic lymphocytic leukemia in 2008, and his brother, who had leukemia and Down syndrome, died at 14 years old.

Larry had not scheduled an annual physical in about 5 years to his detriment. Had he gotten blood work done, a simple CBC would have raised questions, as his white blood cell count was nearly triple what it should be. When he came into my office, Larry felt weak and complained of low energy. He rationalized away his fatigue—he was traveling all the time and putting in too many hours at the office.

Since his white blood cell count was significantly elevated, beyond a common infection, I immediately referred him for further testing to a hematologist-oncologist, a specialist in blood disorders. His lymphocytes were extremely high and neutrophils low, also pointing toward an immune system disorder. With lymphocytes levels as high as his, it was unlikely to be a viral infection. In the face of a markedly elevated WBC, this was likely to be leukemia.

The way we doctors are taught, in general, is to focus all our attention on the disease. That's the usual model. But what about the rest of Larry's sense of well-being? If you recall from Chapter 2 when I introduced Larry, his main goal was to improve his energy levels. Of course, I found the evidence of leukemia to be of immediate concern. Still, I wanted to work with him to strengthen his body and his immune system, boost his metabolism (I found elevated cholesterol, LDL, and triglycerides), and optimize his hormonal function. Raising his testosterone would help him rally against his illness and improve his body's overall function. His hematologist concurred with my plan after the consultation, and he continued to monitor Larry's course.

(continued)

Complete Blood Count

TEST	LOW	HIGH	LARRY'S NUMBERS
WBC (white blood cells)	3.8	10.8	25.5↑*
RBC (red blood cells)	4.2	5.1	4.6
Hemoglobin (protein in red blood cells that carries oxygen)	12	17	14.8
Hematocrit (proportion of total blood volume comprised of red blood cells)	36	51	43.4
Neutrophils, Absolute (a measure of immune function)	1,500	7,800	4,769
Lymphocytes, Absolute (a marker of immune function)	850	3,900	19,457↑*
Neutrophils, %	45	70.9	18.7↓*
Lymphocytes, %	15	45	76.3↑*

* = abnormal, out of range

Measuring red blood cells (RBC) can lead to several different diagnoses, depending on the outcome:

- If they're too big, you're dealing with a nutrient deficiency, and we will want you to ramp up your consumption of vitamin B_{12} and folate.

- If they're too small, it's likely due to an iron deficiency.

- If there are too many of them, you have more oxygen traveling around your bloodstream but you could clot more easily.

- If there are too few of them, you're anemic. You feel run down and weak, with little energy. These symptoms arise over a long period of time, months, or even years and your body compensates, meaning you adjust slowly.

Platelets are another type of cell that's measured in the CBC. Some people may have platelet counts that drop dangerously low, and this decline can be attributed to abnormalities in bone marrow, problems in platelet production or immune system function. Mark L. knew his platelet counts were low, and this is how I managed his care holistically.

PATIENT PROFILE

Mark L.,
AGE 59, REAL ESTATE ATTORNEY

Chief medical concerns: low platelet count, sexual function, general health decline due to aging

Family history: heart attack, migraines, diabetes

Lifestyle: reduced stamina for exercise, problems with sexual function

Goals: improve energy, improve sexual function, manage cholesterol, keep watch on platelet counts

Mark L. was concerned about his health yet skeptical about coming in to see me. Other doctors had told him to beware of any antiaging nonsense or interfering with nature. Aging is inevitable, they said, so he better just get used to it. Mark himself was unfamiliar with testosterone treatment and he was scared to go against the tenets of conventional mainstream medicine.

I spoke to Mark on the phone several times before he came into the office. He did his due diligence and spoke with some of my patients. He took a summer to think it over. He arrived for his first visit with a list of concerns: He was worried about his cholesterol, his weight kept yo-yoing 8 pounds up, 8 pounds down, he couldn't work out without becoming exhausted, and sexual function had recently become an issue. Both he and his wife were struggling with low libido. Depression, arthritis, diabetes,

(continued)

heart attacks, migraines, and cancer ran in his family, and as he was getting older, he wanted to do all he could to lower his risk of becoming ill.
Overall, though, he said he felt okay. Keeping up with the real estate business while raising five kids was a challenge; still, he felt competent as an
attorney and father.

Mark knew his platelet count had been low since the mid-1990s. Then,
he was tested by his primary care doctor, and his bone marrow revealed
that he had what's known as idiopathic thrombocytopenia (ITP). It's
associated with low platelet counts, and platelets are crucial in clotting.
If they're too low, you can hemorrhage, and surgical procedures are risky.
Further tests were ordered to investigate Mark's blood. ITP is more common than you think, and the threat that it poses varies among individuals.
One-third of folks will have platelet counts that continue to drop, and
two-thirds will get better or stay the same. Mark appeared to be in the
majority, having had no problems or precipitous decline in platelet count
in the 12 years since his diagnosis. Still, he was told to avoid aspirin and
ibuprofen (Advil), as these drugs could decrease platelet counts.

His lab data also showed elevated homocysteine despite the fact that
he had been taking folate and medications, which should help lower this
inflammatory marker. He also had high cardiac C-reactive protein (c-CRP)
without any evidence of heart disease. Given these new findings, combined with his low platelet count, he wanted to improve his overall health
and energy. I understood that Mark would be thrilled if his cholesterol
dropped along with his weight.

Complete Blood Count (CBC)

TEST	LOW	HIGH	MARK'S NUMBERS
WBC (white blood cell)	3.8	10.8	4.7
RBC (red blood cell)	4.2	5.1	5.0
Hemoglobin	12	17	16.2
Hematocrit	36	51	46.7
Platelet Count	140	400	132✔*

* = abnormal, out of range

INFLAMMATORY MARKERS
TESTS: CARDIAC-CRP, HOMOCYSTEINE

Whenever there is a rule, there is an exception. I know patients whose cholesterol was within the normal range, yet they would still have a heart attack or a stroke. There had to be other critical pieces of the puzzle that were missing. Cholesterol isn't really the gold standard in predicting cardiovascular disease anymore. Inflammation is also key. In fact, in my opinion, inflammation is the common denominator that links many factors, such as cholesterol, diabetes, dietary issues, and more.

You've heard the stories—your Uncle Ted has cholesterol that's through the roof, but he's in his late eighties and has no evidence of heart disease. Your Aunt Terry, on the other hand, has cholesterol levels that are within range; however, she's been under the care of a cardiologist since her fifties. She's already had one heart attack, and she continues to have angina (chest pains). Her doctor recommended that stents be placed to open up her coronary arteries, because the blockage is likely the cause of her pain and may lead to another heart attack.

How do you explain this? One way may be to look at markers for inflammation.

CARDIAC-CRP. CRP stands for C-reactive protein. The amount of c-CRP in your bloodstream is a direct measure of inflammation in your blood vessels. Specifically, the inflammatory changes are occurring in the endothelium, or the lining of your blood vessels. Why is this important? Increased inflammation in those vessels can contribute to plaque buildup and raise your heart disease and stroke risk.

Measuring c-CRP is a fairly new approach, and it is neither routinely practiced nor well understood. Yet it should be measured in all men, especially those whose LDL levels, lipid profiles, and other risk factors put them on the borderline for requiring a statin in addition to lifestyle modification.

You can have cholesterol numbers within range and still be at high risk for cardiovascular disease if you have elevated c-CRP. When it comes to biomarkers' success at predicting cardiovascular risk, c-CRP is twice as effective as LDL at judging whether or not you'll have a heart attack. Knowing your c-CRP score can help your doctor decide what course of action to take. She may recommend changes to your diet and exercise, or she may prescribe baby aspirin, and possibly a statin, to lower your c-CRP. A large clinical trial known as the Jupiter study showed that rosuvastatin (Crestor) helps bring down c-CRP in subjects who had low to normal cholesterol levels and elevated c-CRPs.

A c-CRP value between 1 and 5 is indicative of cardiovascular risk and signifies inflammation at the level of the endothelium. Generally, guidelines stipulate that a value between 5 and 10 also indicates serious cardiovascular disease. In my experience, however, anything above 5 leads me to suspect that there could also be an infection, inflammation, or injury, that may or may not be directly related to cardiovascular health.

A note of clarification: There is a generalized CRP test that speaks to the whole body. I test *cardiac* CRP, also known as high-sensitivity (hs) CRP, which specifically addresses the health of the lining of the blood vessels, the endothelium.

PATIENT PROFILE

Greg M.,
AGE 49, RESTAURANT OWNER AND CHEF

Chief medical concerns: cardiovascular disease, fatigue, obesity

Family history: high blood pressure, high cholesterol, stroke, congestive heart failure

Lifestyle: reports having no time to exercise; good diet; very stressed; and recently widowed

Goals: better concentration, relief from sadness and anxiety, regain overall health

Ever since he graduated from one of the leading culinary institutes in Paris, Greg M. dreamed of running his own restaurant. In 2007, it became a reality when he opened a French–Asian fusion restaurant.

In 2009, Greg was just shy of 50 and the restaurant was thriving. Yet he was losing his health as a result of being overworked and rundown. He would put in a long workday, head home for dinner, and then drive back to the restaurant where he would stay until around midnight. He also had two young daughters and was a single dad; their mother had died a few months earlier after losing her battle with breast cancer. Recently, his parents moved nearby to help with everything from homework assignments to car-pooling, offering support and guidance while Greg managed his business.

Greg's anxiety and exasperation were evident to me during our first meeting. He was a big guy—6 foot 2 and 220 pounds. He had too much weight around his trunk. Despite eating well (spinach omelettes for breakfast, salad with chicken strips for lunch, whatever he made at the restaurant for dinner, and next-to-no sweets), Greg couldn't seem to get down to his preferred weight of 190, give or take a few pounds. Even though he had taken up running as a hobby at 40, he was now exercise-intolerant and winded after running a couple of miles. If he got home in time before dinner he would lift weights, but this small window was routinely squeezed out of an already too hectic day.

In 2004 and again in 2007, Greg had gotten a cardiac workup since he suffered from heart palpitations and chest tightness; he also had high blood pressure. The tests had revealed nothing out of the ordinary besides a mild murmur (blood rumbling through a heart valve). Regardless, he needed to continue monitoring his cardiac function given his family history. Greg's mother had high blood pressure, congestive heart failure, and a stroke, leaving her wheelchair bound at 60. Greg and his father were both on medi-cations to manage their cholesterol and elevated triglycerides.

When I added the lab data to Greg's story, the most significant finding was a very elevated c-CRP. The inflammatory marker was 4.3, indicating that Greg already had evidence of inflammatory cardiovascular disease.

In addition, Greg's labs revealed significant deficiency in vitamin D at only 24 ng/mL. His total and free testosterone were also very low (273 ng/dL and 48.3 pg/mL, respectively). Coupled with a borderline-high level of luteinizing hormone (LH, the pituitary hormone that stimulates the testes to produce more testosterone), the finding led me to believe he was

(continued)

entering into andropause. We would want to optimize his testosterone levels as quickly as possible to help with his energy and libido as well as his heart function.

Greg wanted to feel more focused, less sad, and less on edge. He wanted to excel at his job, to exercise again, and, most of all, to regain his good health. Greg's main concern was about parenting his young daughters, to always be there for them.

Inflammatory Markers

TEST	LOW	HIGH	GREG'S NUMBER
High-Sensitivity c-CRP	< 1 (optimal)	≥ 1	**4.3↑***

* = abnormal, out of range

HOMOCYSTEINE is an amino acid that damages the lining of the arteries and increases the risk of cardiovascular disease as well as stroke and Alzheimer's disease. Men who have symptoms of atherosclerosis may not have any of the traditional risk factors for heart disease, such as smoking, family history, high LDL cholesterol, or high blood pressure, yet they often have high homocysteine levels. When you don't have enough nutrients, especially B vitamins, homocysteine can rise. Factors that may contribute to these nutrient deficiencies include heavy drinking, poor diet, or poor absorption. Folate (aka vitamin B_9, which occurs in spinach and broccoli) has been thought to help lower homocysteine, yet I've seen many patients on megadoses of folate whose homocysteine levels don't drop. Vitamin B_{12} is another important supplement. For folks who have trouble absorbing vitamin B_{12} in its oral form, it's also available as a medication via injection or nasal spray (Nascobal). The best solution is an improved lifestyle along with a diet chock-full of fruits and vegetables, as well as multiple nutrients, especially those of the B variety.

Keep in mind that if you begin to change your health—working out more and eating better—your metabolic rate may rise, resulting in a bump up in your homocysteine levels. You're using up more nutrients, and your body is under an increased amount of oxidative stress. Given these lifestyle changes, this transient rise in homocysteine is common and expected.

Cedric W.,
AGE 55, CEO

Chief medical concerns: low iron, weight, stress

Family history: obesity, diabetes

Lifestyle: always traveling—tough to stay healthy; outdoorsy; irregular sleep due to stress

Goals: keep up with his on-the-move lifestyle, regain strength

Cedric W. is a man who is always on the move who claims he has a short attention span. He's the CEO for a multinational corporation with work that may take him to Japan on Tuesday, then to Australia on Thursday. It's difficult for him to stay healthy and focused when so much of his life is spent up in the air, his schedule ever-shifting between faraway board meetings and family dinners in Bethesda, Maryland.

Despite his high-octane lifestyle, Cedric didn't drink coffee, tea, or cola. His alcohol intake was about two drinks per week, and even then, he drank only socially. His sleep was generally good, except when he was stressed. Then he would find himself watching a lot of reruns instead of getting any shut-eye. He did his best to lead an active lifestyle—rock climbing, golfing, running, and spending some quality time with the rowing machine at any chance he got.

Still, weight was always an issue. It was for everybody in his family, too—mom, dad, brother. His father was overweight and diabetic, while his mother had passed away in her early seventies due to complications after breaking her hip. In 2005, Cedric underwent gastric bypass surgery. Soon thereafter, he dropped 100 pounds.

When he came into my office, Cedric was 200 pounds and 6 foot 1. I remember him looking lean and fairly healthy, though I noticed he was very pale. On the phone he had said he was doing well overall. Six months prior to coming to see me, he had gotten blood work done, which indicated that

(continued)

his iron levels were too low. His primary care doctor prescribed supplements, though, sometimes Cedric forgot to take his pills.

It turns out that the gastric bypass was preventing Cedric's body from absorbing not only iron but also B_{12} and folate. This was reflected in his blood work. My testing revealed elevated homocysteine and low iron, hemoglobin, hematocrit, mean corpuscular volume (MCV), and mean corpuscular hemoglobin (MCH), all measures related to red blood cells and characteristic of anemia. Cedric had never had a colonoscopy and considering the finding of anemia on his CBC (page 58), I wanted to rule out cancer immediately. You may bleed internally from cancer in your gastrointestinal tract, so your body loses its iron stores. I sent him to a gastrointestinal specialist to investigate further.

Cedric was looking for a way to keep up with his lifestyle and regain his strength, some of which he felt he lost after the gastric bypass procedure. That meant he would need a highly practical and time-efficient approach that would lead him to improve his health as he traveled the world.

Inflammatory Markers

TEST	LOW	HIGH	CEDRIC'S NUMBER
Homocysteine	0	9	12.3↑*

* = abnormal, out of range

BONE STUDIES
TESTS: BONE DENSITY, BODY COMPOSITION

Compared to women, men usually are at greater risk for heart disease at a younger age, beginning in their late thirties. This is where medicine's focus has been. The reverse is true for osteoporosis (bone loss), so most of the focus for this disorder associated with aging is on women. Women, due in part to lower levels of testosterone, manifest bone loss starting in their forties, about 10 years prior to the average male. Men, though, do catch up. In my family, it was my father and his side of the family who had osteoporosis.

The reality is about 25 percent of men and women will develop osteoporosis, hip fractures, or the curved spine known as a buffalo hump. I frequently see men staring down, shaped as an inverted U, presumably due to irreversible osteoporosis. Only recently, however, has the Endocrine Society recommended that men get bone density screenings, lending credence to the notion that men also get osteoporosis with age. Guidelines now say that men should be screened at age 70, but why wait that long? Men should have baseline bone density scans just like women, with an initial scan in their thirties to determine whether they're already at risk of developing osteopenia, denoting abnormally low bone density. Osteopenia often leads to osteoporosis if action isn't taken. In fact, I have detected bone loss in men in their thirties due to an overactive parathyroid gland that would have gone undetected for years. There are also men who, similar to women, never built adequate bone in their youth, and already manifest risk at 30 or 40. Why wait until building bone is a challenge and fractures are more common as men reach 70 and beyond?

PATIENT PROFILE

Marvin Lagstein,
AGE 67, DENTIST AND BUSINESS OWNER

Chief medical concerns: defying his genetics and not succumbing to the disorders of aging as many of his relatives had

Family history: diabetes, cardiovascular disease

Lifestyle: serious marathon runner; near-impeccable diet; too many supplements

Goals: be well enough to dance at his youngest daughter's wedding

Marvin Lagstein knew his family history, and he knew it wasn't good. Many of his relatives had diabetes and heart disease; some died at a

(continued)

young age. Marvin was the only child of two Holocaust survivors who lived into their eighties, so he also knew something about resilience. In order to stay healthy, he had taken up running when he was young. By age 65, he had run in more than 25 marathons and routinely jogged 10 miles every other day. Our exercise physiologist, Steven, and I knew Marvin was doing damage to his body the first time we saw him.

Given Marvin's appearance, you might have guessed that he had a chronic illness. We tried to tag team him, telling him that he should lighten up on the running and focus instead on stretching or resistance training. He would play it cute: "I can't hear you. There's static on the line." He thought he looked fine. But there was real fear behind his denial. He was having night sweats and suffered from high blood pressure and some reduction in energy. Most surprising to Marvin, given his exercise and eating habits, was his weight gain. His pants were getting tighter around his waist.

Of course, it helped that Marvin was trying to eat right and had been a vegetarian for a quarter century. Yet, with that much stress on his musculoskeletal system, he still had an emaciated look about him that made him appear weak, as if he were wasting away from some chronic disease. He wasn't building bone. In fact, with his relentless running, he was tearing down whatever bone he had, actually causing stress fractures. Too much of anything, including exercise, can be harmful to your health, and such was the case with Marvin.

I finally cajoled him into getting a bone density scan. A dual-energy x-ray absorptiometry (DEXA) scan can measure your bone density. If your doctor requests a body composition scan (requires specialized software) in addition, this test will show the breakdown of fat mass and lean muscle. With a DEXA scan, you'll be exposed to a minimal amount of radiation, about one-tenth that of a chest x-ray. That's less than the amount of radiation you get going through airport security.

Marvin had never had a bone density scan before, and he was scared. Yet knowing his family's history, Marvin underwent the DEXA scan so he could take action to prevent future bone loss. The results of the scan revealed stress fractures and osteoporosis. They also showed his T-score, which was calculated by comparing Marvin's bone density to what's normally expected of men in their late twenties who are in peak health. His T-score showed he was at significant risk—meaning brittleness, fractures, breaks—in the future.

When Marvin began my program, he had a second wife 20 years his junior and a daughter who was ready to start kindergarten. When the time came, he wanted to be there at his youngest daughter's wedding—not just watching but dancing in great health.

Marvin's Bone Density Scan

	LUMBAR SPINE	FEMORAL NECK		TOTAL HIP		FOREARM	
		Right	Left	Right	Left	Right	Left
Normal							
Osteopenia		X		X	X	X	X
Osteoporosis	X		X				

Even if you're not in the medical profession, chances are you've heard of EKG, BP, and BMI. Body mass index is a measure that uses your weight and height to determine obesity and can serve as a predictor for diseases like diabetes and hypertension. Yet despite its widespread use, especially in studies involving large populations, BMI is not actually the best measure for determining body composition. In fact, much like looks, an "attractive" BMI can be deceiving.

For example, someone who is 5 feet 9 inches and weighs 185 pounds is considered to be obese by BMI standards. It turns out that this person may actually have only 8 percent body fat (i.e., he's got muscle on him, and muscle weighs more than fat). On the other end of the spectrum, another person of the same height who weighs 165 pounds—the recommended or healthy weight for someone 5 foot 9—may be at 35 percent body fat, most of which is located above his belt buckle. This person gets an A+ on the BMI rating scale, but he's actually fairly unhealthy.

The thing about BMI is that its scope is too simplistic. It doesn't differentiate between the three components that make up the human body: bone, fat mass, and lean muscle.

Other measures of body composition are more sensitive to the individual, including waist-to-height ratio (WtHR), which studies have shown to be significantly better at predicting your risk of developing hypertension and diabetes. Even a seven-site skinfold test is more reliable, though subjective in execution, than BMI in the short term.

I like our patients to get a body composition scan, which measures body fat percentage and lean muscle tissue. The procedure is painless and easy, taking only about 15 minutes to complete. As previously described, it can be done with the DEXA bone density if the software is available. You would have to pay for the test out of pocket, as insurance providers consider this a "vanity" test, when in fact it is one of the best predictors of health available.

Greg M., whom you met on page 64, underwent a body composition along with his DEXA (bone density) scan before coming in for his initial health analysis with me and my team. Not only was his total percent body fat above what I would like to see for a man under 50, but the percent body fat around his middle was even 2.5 percentage points higher. Ideally, you will want to aim to have the percent body fat of your trunk be less than your overall percent body fat. I helped Greg eat more regularly and cut back on those spinach omelettes to eliminate his risk of gout because his uric acid level was high. I also wanted him to up his resistance training to build more muscle. You can read more about the recommended types of exercise in Chapter 7. Another component that would help Greg to get his body fat percentage back within an optimal range is an adjustment of his hormone levels. Chapter 4 will introduce you to the different kinds of hormones and give you an appreciation for why each is vital to your health.

Greg's Body Composition Scan

OVERALL BODY FAT	30.1%↑*
REGIONAL BREAKDOWN:	
Fat in the trunk	32.6%↑*
Fat in the left arm	23.5%
Fat in the left leg	29.8%
Fat in the right arm	20.0%
Fat in the right leg	27.5%

* = abnormal, out of range

AND THAT'S NOT ALL

Now I've added another layer to your personal health metrics. Along with your personal history, family history, and lifestyle, your lab stats add a degree of precision and objectivity to your story. Hormones are another critical piece of your puzzle. You already know that testosterone has a major impact on your metabolic function, and that a hormonal imbalance underlies many health problems. Next I'll add still another significant component to complement the constellation you've already gathered: the major hormones you'll want to know that affect every aspect of your vitality.

CHAPTER 4

THE HORMONE TESTS

Putting together the pieces of your puzzle

I first met Dr. Comite in Memphis at a conference of the American Nutraceutical Association. She did a lecture on her work with andropausal men, a term I had not heard before. In her case study of a man 18 years my junior, I immediately recognized myself. I decided to get my own evaluation.

I was surprised across the board. I never had such a thorough evaluation before. I'd never had such a real collaborator on my health before. I found out I had low testosterone, which I figured was the case. What I didn't expect, however, was also having an underactive thyroid. I realized that in 15 years of annual checkups, my thyroid had never been included in the basic testing.

—**STEPHEN HEFLER,** MD, age 68, pediatrician

A t almost 70 years of age, Dr. Hefler recognized that he was facing challenges with his health that began more than 20 years earlier. Thyroid testing had not been included in his lab data, which isn't necessarily surprising. Typical lab testing for an annual visit with your primary physician is generally limited to basic metabolic tests, including urinalysis, fasting glucose, lipid panel, complete blood count (CBC), and a kidney and liver profile. A hormone panel, except for thyroid-stimulating hormone (TSH), is often not ordered. This is troubling, as hormones have a tremendous impact on metabolism and play a vital role in sustaining health.

The thyroid, for instance, is a gland at the base of your neck that is overactive or underactive in some individuals. Dr. Hefler's thyroid was underactive, a condition known as hypothyroidism. Symptoms include weight gain, depression, fatigue, aches and pains, constipation, and swelling of the extremities. Dr. Hefler experienced several of these and other symptoms: He noticed a general fogginess to his thoughts, and he was losing his eyebrows.

Frequently, doctors will ask me: "Can you look at this thyroid?" My answer is: "Not without knowing more about this individual." I don't look at the thyroid in isolation. It is not a single organ separate from the human who houses it. I prefer to—actually I *need* to—know about the whole person. The thyroid is responsible for a whole host of communications that requires interaction between your brain, your heart, your bones, and more. A personal medical history will illuminate signs and symptoms like Dr. Hefler's. Later in this chapter, you'll meet another patient, Ethan H., whose mother had thyroid disease—an example of how family history can contribute to a diagnosis as well. Lifestyle factors, especially exposure to high stress situations, may also contribute to changes in thyroid hormone production. Finally, because a chain of events contributes to hypothyroidism, a deeper investigation is needed using a more complete blood test called a thyroid panel.

As you saw with the metabolic tests, your hormone tests will help us get a more complete picture of who you are overall. Your hormones are critical pieces of your health puzzle. Knowing whether your hormone levels are within range is extremely useful, yet this information is often overlooked, unknown, and undervalued by doctors. Hormones speak to the whole body health and, paired with other biomarkers, give insight into the disorders of aging, such as heart attack, stroke, diabetes, and osteoporosis. As I've explained, my interest in hormones and the field of endocrinology began with my exposure to young children going through puberty well before their 10th birthday. Later I continued my research in adults, also undergoing hormonal interventions that allowed me unique insights into the mind and body.

My clinical research base gave me an appreciation for how nuanced aging really is. I saw maturation in each decade, which is very different from the transition from childhood to adulthood. We may stop growing upward, yet our bodies and our minds continue to evolve, and hormones shape these changes.

Although the field of endocrinology has long been established, doctors, even endocrinologists, have traditionally ignored hormones when evaluating a man's health. Women's health dominated the discipline ever since menopause came out of the proverbial closet in the early 1980s: Women no longer thought of themselves as old after they went through "the change"; after all, many of them had waited until their late thirties and early forties to start families.

What's more, in contrast to men's symptoms of midlife hormone change, women mostly exhibit easily recognizable, physical signs beginning 5 or 10 years prior to menopause. They have hot flashes and disrupted sleep patterns; intercourse becomes painful, periods become irregular, and urinary tract infections occur more frequently. Men's symptoms are often much more vague and elusive. Two common complaints I hear from male patients are low energy and persistent fatigue. At times, men also mention facial flushing and body sweats. Low libido is currently cited as the most frequent complaint associated with low testosterone. Erectile dysfunction is another common sign, but because this symptom is often due to other health problems it is harder to link to hormonal changes. In response to these complaints, many doctors may offer pat wisdom and temporary fixes. They say the energy drop is "just something you're going to have to get used to" while writing out a prescription for Viagra, Cialis, or Levitra.

Looking at hormones in men is a new phenomenon. It wasn't until recently, when the "Do you have low T?" television ads first aired, that testosterone decline with age began to be taken seriously. The antecedents to this campaign date back to the 1990s when the Department of Defense put millions ($840 million by 1999) into breast cancer research, and some men, particularly those in Congress, were outraged. There

Traditional Medicine Is Slow to Change

It will take time before mainstream medicine appreciates Precision Medicine, where collecting personal health metrics on each patient is commonplace and disease prevention is our main goal. The conflicts I face in changing the way the medical community thinks about aging remind me of struggles faced by my colleague and former US surgeon general, the late C. Everett Koop, MD (or Chick, as he was nicknamed), when he began assembling a pediatric surgery department at the Children's Hospital of Philadelphia in the 1940s and 1950s after pioneering several surgical procedures there. The field got its official start a few years earlier under William E. Ladd, MD, at Children's Hospital Boston, though Dr. Koop was right on the heels of its creation. Most people in the medical community still saw children as little adults when in fact their systems are much different. For instance, a 7-year-old's brain is not just a miniature version of an adult brain. There is a tremendous amount of growth yet to come in the brain's size and plasticity as well as in the creation and strengthening of neuronal connections. It follows, then, that surgical procedures would have to account for all this. We've made significant progress. As of 2003, there were more than 30 training programs in pediatric surgery in the United States, many of which prepare doctors in subspecialties like neonatal surgery and fetal surgery. Today, we often take this field for granted, whereas its acceptance by the medical community was anything but easy.

were ads all over Washington, DC, announcing that men weren't getting their fair share of funding for prostate cancer. Soon, there were efforts to increase funding for prostate cancer research. In the '90s, scientists identified a protein known as prostate-specific antigen (PSA) as a marker of the cancer and testing became more widespread. In a very short period, it seems, we have witnessed a sea of change in appreciation in men's health. I have seen that the medical community and my fellow endocrinologists have begun to appreciate that the production of hormones are vital to overall health.

Hormones clearly are crucial to a man's health. Hormones are protective in a multitude of ways. There's a relationship between the decline in hormones of various types and diseases such as diabetes, heart disease, reduced bone density, depression—you name it, the list goes on and on. The research has begun to support clinical findings, and that's where the field of andrology is going. While there is much yet to learn, you can take advantage of this new science today. I'm doing it in my practice, and other doctors are starting to as well. In the pages that follow, I'll take a look at each of these hormones that are so important to the proper function of your body and how they are measured. They include:

- The sex steroid hormones testosterone, dehydroepiandrosterone (DHEA), estradiol (E_2), and dihydrotestosterone (DHT)

- Thyroid-stimulating hormone (TSH), which is produced by the pituitary gland to tell the thyroid gland to release thyroid hormones, such as free thyroid hormones known as T3 and T4, into the bloodstream

- Insulin and cortisol, which relate to carbohydrate metabolism and stress

- Insulin-like growth factor 1 (IGF-1), an indirect measure of human growth hormone (HGH)

- Vitamin D, which is indeed a hormone, despite its misleading moniker

- Prostate-specific antigen (PSA), a protein associated with testosterone and DHT

THE HORMONE TESTS: TESTOSTERONE, DHEA, DHT, ESTRADIOL, AND PSA

A simple blood test is used to measure levels of each of these hormones.

TESTOSTERONE, as you've learned, is critically important. When the negative feedback loop involving hormones of the brain and testes—specifically gonadotropin-releasing hormone (GnRH), luteinizing hormone (LH), and testosterone—isn't working as it should, less T is circulated through your body, and free T levels drop. As you age, a host of factors may contribute to this decline. Total testosterone, less than 350 ng/dL is considered low, while less than 280 ng/dL is associated with symptoms. Still, most endocrinologists would recommend repeating the test again to be certain it is not an exception. For optimal functioning, free T should fall between 150 and 250 pg/mL. Calculated free testosterone should be greater than 80 pg/mL.

I want to point out that while the free T value is good to use as a rough indicator to target as a range, in general, it is not enough. Most important, however, is not the exact number but, rather, your clinical response. Some men might do just fine with a free T of 130 pg/mL: the symptoms of low T completely ameliorated, sex is good, fat around the middle has diminished, energy has recovered, and more. Yet another man, with a free T of 200 pg/mL, still notes difficulty with erections, depression, fatigue, some improved symptoms, maybe 5 on a scale of 1 to 10.

A precursor to testosterone, DHEA is responsible for the synthesis of testosterone. DHEA levels also begin to wane as men hit their thirties, affecting testosterone production. As men reach their forties, the balance starts shifting from a less androgenic state to one that includes more estrogen. It can undermine male sexual function because estrogen competes with testosterone at the receptor binding sites. There is also an increase in sex hormone-binding globulin (SHBG) secreted by the liver. You're probably thinking that this is becoming quite a mouthful of acronyms. Don't worry; there's no quiz at the end of the book! The important thing to keep in mind is that SHBG binds to testosterone, which ties up the hormone, making testosterone unable to target its receptor sites and perform its role. And that means less testosterone is available to your body.

What's more, as men gain weight during their forties (due in part due to the fall in T), the fat that replaces muscle levies an additional cost to the body. Within fat is an enzyme called aromatase that converts testosterone into estradiol (or E_2), a type of estrogen. Men who are overweight often have increased levels of aromatase. This may lead to elevated estrogen, which interferes with T binding to receptors in the body. The other breakdown product of testosterone is the androgen dihydrotestosterone, or DHT for short. This relationship is a little less linear. Some men will have a high level of DHT and low T, meaning that much of their free testosterone is getting broken down, whereas others may have low levels of DHT and adequate T. Again, this association is highly individual.

It's especially important to measure DHT because high levels can elevate PSA, which is produced in the testicles and usually remains below 4 nanograms per milliliter (ng/mL). If PSA increases, it's generally for one of three reasons: (1) acute prostatitis, which is an infection in the prostate; (2) benign prostatic hyperplasia (BPH), where the prostate is enlarged, which happens in many men and can be driven by high levels of DHT; or (3) prostate cancer, which produces a slow, steady rise of PSA. So therein lies the confusion. If your doctor thinks your elevated PSA is due to an infection, she can culture the prostate fluid and treat it with antibiotics. Because doctors expect to find multiple bugs living in the prostatic fluid, however, they often skip the culture and treat with a broad-spectrum antibiotic. Your doctor may also look at the percent free PSA, a portion of the total, which can sometimes distinguish between a benign condition and potential malignancy. You're usually in the clear if the percent free is high. Later you'll meet a patient of mine who had a high PSA, and we had to play detective to get to the root cause.

Ed H.,
AGE 47, ACCOUNTANT

Chief medical concerns: low testosterone, andropause

Family history: arthritis, sclerosis

Lifestyle: 4 months of bad habits; 8 months of eating right, getting enough sleep, and leading spin classes

Goals: regain strength, prevent disorders of aging

If it's true that the only things certain in life are death and taxes, then as an accountant, Ed H. knew this better than anybody. In the months leading up to April 15, he would sleep in his office, alternating between eating nothing and nothing but takeout. He rarely exercised, let alone slept. When he did, sleep apnea was a problem. Once taxes were over, however, he would get away to Fire Island where he ran a spinning class and worked out incessantly. Lifestyle-wise, the other three seasons acted like a buffer against Ed's poor habits and tremendous stress during the winter months.

When he came into my office for the first time, Ed looked very trim and athletic. It appeared he took care of himself. I was surprised to learn, then, while conducting his physical examination, that he had limited range of motion in his right shoulder. He reported that he had arthritis and sustained two tendon tears. In the past few years, he had lost 15 to 20 pounds, partly because he couldn't lift weights as a result of the injuries. He also had had a hip replacement in 2009 and was advised to take 2 years off from running. He switched to cycling and did yoga and Pilates. Ed had a family history of arthritis, and his mother suffered from sclerosis. He had begun taking L-arginine to maximize his workouts and help build muscle (more on that in Chapter 8).

But why was Ed losing so much muscle in the first place? Yes, he had

(continued)

had injuries, but he was also exercising a lot. Ed's labs revealed that his total and free testosterone levels were very low, 555 ng/dL and 87 pg/mL, respectively. This helped to explain his low libido and also accounted for his weight loss. Without testosterone, his body wasn't able to put on lean muscle as he had in prior years. Looking closer, lab results showed that Ed's LH was high, indicating that he was in andropause. This is uncommon in a man as young as Ed, but it does happen. I've seen men enter andropause as early as their late thirties. Because Ed was so young, I had to make a decision about how to bring his testosterone levels back up to optimal levels. As for Ed, he wanted to regain his physical and psychological fortitude and avoid illness as he aged.

Hormone Panel

TESTS	LOW	HIGH	ED'S NUMBERS
Cortisol, Total	<4	>16	19.9↑*
Testosterone, Total	700	900	555↓*
Testosterone, Free	130	190	86.6↓*
Dihydrotestosterone	25	75	56
Luteinizing Hormone (LH)	1.5	9.3	11.3↑*
Estradiol, High-Sensitivity	10	40	36†
DHEA Sulfate	350	500	45↓*
PSA, Total	0	4	0.4
IGF-1	<100	>350	195

* = abnormal, out of range

†Ed's estradiol was at the upper range of the spectrum, likely in part because his testosterone was being converted via aromatase. Recall that estradiol levels may increase as men age.

If you are diagnosed with low T, your doctor may prescribe synthetic testosterone in one of various forms that she thinks is best suited to your case. Testosterone is available as injections, gels applied to the skin, or patches worn on the skin (sometimes the scrotum).

Testosterone therapy must be closely monitored by your doctor through ongoing blood tests to manage possible side effects. Some of the common ones are as follows:

- Breast tingling, which may evolve to breast enlargement

- Testicular shrinkage

- Decrease in HDL cholesterol

- Increased red blood cell count

- Decreased sperm count

As with any intervention, even aspirin, there are upsides and downsides. Left unchecked, testosterone therapy may raise your risk of developing certain conditions such as polycythemia (thickened blood) or gynecomastia (enlarged breasts). Thicker blood may result because the testosterone increases the production of red blood cells, and if too much testosterone converts to estrogen, you may get nipple tingling as well as breast tissue. One of the reasons you might see this tissue is that 70 percent of boys, as they go through puberty, can develop either unilateral or bilateral breast tissue that later goes away. If you were one of those boys, you may be more likely to experience breast development during testosterone therapy because perhaps the tissue never completely went away and is now being stimulated. Correctly balanced by a doctor, the benefits of treatment with T should well outweigh these risks.

Topical treatment is the most common hormone therapy available for men. First, your doctor will have to test your T levels (see Getting Better Blood Work on page 93); then you have to identify what your doctor is comfortable prescribing. I almost always use testosterone injections because they are most effective and there is no risk of transference to others via skin contact. For men who have not yet gone through andropause, I like to use human chorionic gonadotropin (hCG). (Note: This is not available in topical form, and I only prescribe injectible hCG.) The benefit is that hCG spurs your body to produce its own testosterone, which is a good thing. Once again, I'm a firm believer in working with the body. If I can get your organs to do what they should do well, that's the ideal solution. There are also data that suggest there are biological benefits to keeping your testes active as long possible, the idea being that the longer the body is able to reproduce, the greater the chances that you'll live longer. In fact, research shows that women who can still conceive later in life—in their forties and beyond—have increased longevity.

The most important factor is the way your body and mind respond to any intervention, including testosterone and hCG (human chorionic gonadotropin). Your response to T can only be measured using your own indicators, signs, and symptoms. This is true for many reasons. You may absorb T differently from other men, metabolize it faster or slower; your particular makeup dictates your response.

It's important to remember that the breakdown products of testosterone, estradiol, and DHT may also need to be managed with medication should you begin treatment. As you increase T, there may be an uptick in either or both of these hormones. Both estradiol and DHT are frequently overlooked; however, they are two very important biomarkers that should be monitored as long as you're receiving hormone therapy. Remember, too, you should establish what your baseline levels are before beginning treatment.

THYROID FUNCTION TESTS. The thyroid gland controls how quickly the body uses energy and makes proteins; it also controls how sensitive the body is to other hormones. The two hormones it makes, free thyroid 3 (T3) and free thyroid 4 (T4), regulate metabolism and affect the growth as well as rate of function of many other systems in the body. Someone who has *hypothyroidism,* like Dr. Hefler, doesn't produce enough thyroid hormone. When this occurs, levels of thyroid-stimulating hormone—the hormone that stimulates the thyroid to work harder—are often high. *Hyperthyroidism* is the opposite condition: The body produces too much thyroid hormone, and TSH levels are usually low. Think of it as a seesaw— one goes up, so the other goes down.

Still, this action-reaction way of looking at things is too linear. There's no way I can tell if an individual has a deficient thyroid by looking only at TSH levels, though, as I mentioned earlier, TSH is typically the only hormone that's ordered in blood tests. Normal TSH levels can range from 0.4 to 5.5 milli-international units per liter (mIU/L). That's more than a tenfold difference. Measuring T3 and T4 is necessary to figure out whether the thyroid is malfunctioning. If T3 and T4 are elevated, the brain won't send a signal to create more thyroid, so TSH will be low.

Conversely, if T3 and T4 are low, the brain will send a signal through the pituitary to produce more thyroid, so TSH will be high. Measurements can vary in several ways even beyond what I've outlined here, and there is no way to reach a diagnosis without all these values. I've identified optimal values and target ranges; still, it's the relationships between these numbers that are most important.

Your TSH would have to be abnormal, say 7 mIU/L, for the doctor to measure actual thyroid output, T3 and T4. I've seen cases, however, where TSH came in at an apparently "normal" 4 mIU/L, yet T3 was 1.8 mIU/L. To be functional, it needs to be at least 3 mIU/L. This relationship between TSH and T3 shows that the pituitary is telling the thyroid to work, except the thyroid isn't listening. If you have symptoms, identify contributing lifestyle factors and know your family history, then share them with your doctor. Together you can put the puzzle pieces into place.

PATIENT PROFILE

Ethan B.,
AGE 39, HIGH SCHOOL PRINCIPAL

Chief medical concerns: hypothyroidism

Family history: thyroid problems, obesity, cardiovascular disease

Lifestyle: poor diet, very little exercise, too much caffeine, diminished sexual function

Goals: lose weight, gain energy

Ever since his teens, Ethan B. was never comfortable with his body, so much so that he hesitated to get into relationships with women, fearful of physical rejection. Despite being a member of a gym, he rarely went. As a high school principal, Ethan worked long hours, meeting with students and staff during the day and attending board meetings, the spring musical, or Friday night football games at night. He fueled his body with caffeine, which gave him heart palpitations.

(continued)

There were several reasons Ethan couldn't lose weight, and his lab numbers helped to explain his personal history. Ethan had borderline hypothyroidism. This situation likely went undetected because his TSH was still within range. His T3 and T4 were low, however, which indicated that his metabolic rate was sluggish. The mitochondria, or the energy producers in cells, were not working as efficiently. His elevated homocysteine indicated a nutrient deficiency. What's more, his hemoglobin A1c was borderline though within range at 5.6 percent (5.7 percent is prediabetic). His blood sugar was too low after fasting overnight, revealing reactive hypoglycemia. When you're hypoglycemic, it triggers the release of cortisol, and cortisol promotes the storage of carbs as fat. This is what was happening to Ethan. Finally, underlying it all, Ethan's total and free testosterone were very low, 253 ng/dL and 49 pg/mL, respectively. This made it difficult for Ethan to develop lean muscle. Unlike fat, muscles engage in metabolism even at rest. So the more muscles you have, the more calories you burn. Other hormones that were low included Ethan's DHEA and his DHT.

Ethan's family history put him at greater risk for disease. His father and brother were heavy, and his father also had high blood pressure and cardiovascular disease. His mother recently found a lump on her thyroid and her doctors gave her a medication to suppress thyroid function. As I said earlier, this was a critical piece of information when it came to diagnosing Ethan's hypothyroidism.

When he came to my office, Ethan was overweight and clearly uncomfortable in his own skin. That said, he was excited about our recommendations and eager to make improvements. He had a good spirit about him. He wanted to have one last blowout party before he began any treatment.

Ethan's hope was to lose weight, gain energy, and travel without feeling worn out.

Thyroid Panel

TESTS	LOW	HIGH	ETHAN'S NUMBERS
TSH	0.4	5.5	1.95
T3, Free	2.3	4.2	2.0✔*
T4, Free	0.8	1.8	0.6✔*

* = abnormal, out of range

CORTISOL. Cortisol is a stress hormone secreted by the adrenal glands that impacts your blood sugar level. Stress, whether it involves angry co-workers or a three-car pileup, raises your cortisol level. If cortisol is too high, this negatively impacts your sugar metabolism, causing you to store energy as fat. This makes you gain weight around the middle. During periods of particularly high stress, you may experience burnout, at which point cortisol drops below optimal levels. Generally, we like to see cortisol between 6 and 10 micrograms per deciliter (mg/dL) in the morning, when it's at its peak. The following story describes an actor who was experiencing anxiety both on and off camera, noticing that his health was suffering as a result.

PATIENT PROFILE

Noah N.,
AGE 60, ACTOR

Chief medical concerns: high cortisol, low testosterone

Family history: ulcers, coronary artery disease, high blood pressure, psychiatric illness

Lifestyle: heavy drinker, smoker, stressed and frazzled, good diet, minimal exercise (Pilates)

Goals: manage anxiety, boost libido, quit smoking, lose weight

Noah N. was on a transcontinental flight when he had a sort of epiphany. Noah had just turned 60 and was starring in a new summer action film. In an industry whose home base is Hollywood, where a premium is placed on looking good no matter the means, Noah wanted more of a wholesale transformation—"Project Noah," he was calling it. He thought it would take about 12 months before he was once again in control of his own health. He had to learn to take care of himself on a daily basis now that he couldn't rely on his body to bounce back after every high-profile screening. Even though he ate well and did Pilates occasionally, he had

(continued)

been noticing some changes in his health: an extra inch or two added to his girth, sleep deprivation, flagging sex drive, and a nicotine addiction (25 cigarettes per day) that he couldn't seem to kick. Most importantly, he had always been anxious. Yet he figured that by 60, he should have mellowed out. Often, he drank to help quiet his mind. He didn't like the way antianxiety meds made him feel, so he didn't take any. Even though he looked great for his age, he felt his mood and habits wearing on his health.

His family's history was peppered with coronary artery disease, high blood pressure, and psychiatric illness. Both his parents passed away in their midseventies, and his two sisters suffered from recurring ulcers. Noah himself had had a duodenal ulcer and persistent *H. pylori* (a kind of stomach bacteria) flare-ups, though both were resolved in his twenties.

Noah first came to my office in the spring of 2010. Consistent with his self-reports of anxiety, his cortisol levels were also extremely high, likely a result of the pressures of having a job in the public eye. What's more, Noah's testosterone, both total and free, was very low. His LH was high, though, signaling that he was going through andropause.

"Project Noah" was gearing up with goals that included dropping the extra pounds around his middle, losing his nicotine habit, recovering his libido, and, most importantly, managing his anxiety.

Hormone Panel

TESTS	LOW	HIGH	NOAH'S NUMBERS
Cortisol, Total	<4	>16	24.4↑*
Testosterone, Total	700	900	309↓*
Testosterone, Free	130	190	49↓*
Testosterone, %Free	1	2.7	0.46
Dihydrotestosterone	25	75	42
Luteinizing Hormone (LH)	1.5	9.3	7.2†
Estradiol, High-Sensitivity	10	40	15
DHEA Sulfate	350	500	36↓*
PSA, Total	0	4	0.6
IGF-1	<100	>350	104

* = abnormal, out of range

†It is important to look at Noah's LH in relation to his T. Because 7.2 is at the higher end of the reference range, he is likely to be in andropause. In my experience, an LH higher than 5 is a reliable indicator of andropause.

VITAMIN D. It's called a vitamin, but it's really a hormone. Vitamin D is present in many cells throughout the body, and data suggest it plays a role in everything from cardiovascular health to the immune system. Vitamin D is responsible for getting the important bone builders— calcium and phosphorus—to the places in the body where they can help bone remineralize. It's also been shown to help brain function and facilitate oxygen absorption. The Institute of Medicine recommends that folks 70 and younger get 600 international units (IU) of vitamin D daily. That number rises to 800 IU for the over-70 crowd. In general, I recommend supplements for my patients, as I aim for D levels that reach 60 to 80 IU. It's not so clear, however, what amounts you should be taking and what role vitamin D has once you get beyond the levels that I presume would be optimal level.

A study in the journal *Nutrition* from 2010 estimates that 42 percent of Americans are deficient in vitamin D; our diet, alcohol consumption (with too much alcohol, the liver cannot process vitamin D effectively), and too little time spent exposed to the sun, all contribute to our subpar levels. Good natural sources of vitamin D include milk, yogurt, and other dairy products as well as green leafy veggies such as broccoli and kale. A no-calorie option is stepping outside in the sun for 20 to 60 minutes each day (do use sunscreen). In my experience though, D doesn't really increase all that much with sun exposure. And remember, in northern climates, the sun is effective as a vitamin D source only seasonally—in late spring, summer, and early fall; it isn't strong enough during the winter.

Usually, I recommend vitamin D supplementation as well. Supplementation is available for both vitamin D_2 (ergocalciferol) and vitamin D_3 (cholecalciferol); vitamin D_2 requires a prescription, while vitamin D_3 can be purchased over the counter. The reason I mention both is that some people have trouble absorbing vitamin D_3 and often find the prescription form more effective.

Widespread deficiency is something I see in my clinical practice, and I prescribe vitamin D for the vast majority of my patients. In fact, too little vitamin D may have played a major role in the cardiovascular health of a patient of mine, Tony N., contributing to his stroke.

PATIENT PROFILE

Tony N.,
AGE 53, RETIRED ARMY GENERAL

Chief medical concerns: stroke

Family history: cardiovascular disease, hyperlipidemia

Lifestyle: tried to be healthy, but his diabetes and low hormones
(namely testosterone and vitamin D) were undermining his best efforts

Goals: recover from stroke, regain energy, lose weight, gain muscle

Sometimes people come to see me when they're on the cliff's edge, about
ready to fall. The minute I hear their story, it's as if I can see a piece of
paper taped to their backs saying, "heart attack" or "stroke." It's that
obvious they're headed for trouble soon. For some, it is imminent, unless
we stage an intervention. Such was the case with Tony N.

With Tony, there was only a sliver of time—a day and a half—between
when his results were available and when we were scheduled to chat on
the phone. Before I could call him, however, his wife called us to say he'd
been admitted to the hospital after suffering a stroke. His stay there
lasted 2 weeks. He had lower extremity and upper extremity weakness
and difficulties with activities of daily living; the right side of his face
had gone flat.

Once I received Tony's lab results, I knew he was in serious trouble,
which is why I tried to schedule the call with him as quickly as possible.
Many of his hormones—testosterone (total and free), IGF-1, T3—all were
low. His PSA, on the other hand, was high, warranting further investigation.

At 53, with a high LH and low testosterone, it looked as though Tony
was in andropause. He was on the younger end of the spectrum, yet we
had to consider that this was the case given his symptoms. In some
instances, a man is not yet in andropause, though the brain responds to
the low T, albeit transiently. When the pituitary recognizes that testosterone is low, pulses of LH are released. It acts like a drummer beating on the

testes with LH to try to get them to increase testosterone production. Since the lab tests only measure one point in time, I may have caught Tony when LH was at a high point, trying to encourage the testes to produce more testosterone. Repeat testing and tracking his results over time would give me a clearer picture on his hormonal function, indicating whether he was in andropause.

Of note, vitamin D was well below optimal levels. If it had been low over a long enough period of time, it is possible that insufficient D could play a role in contributing to the cardiovascular issues that led to his stroke.

There is research to support this hypothosis. Tony also said he had difficulty maintaining erections and no longer experienced morning erections—explainable, given his low T in combination with a finding of insulin resistance and troubling cholesterol levels. The pudendal arteries (which are important in engorging the penis during sex) were likely blocked by plaque, due to inflammation in the presence of high cholesterol and sugar. This made his bloodflow sluggish. The pudendal arteries are one-quarter of the size of coronary arteries, which is why erectile dysfunction is commonly thought of as a predictor of cardiac disease. Additionally, his family history of cardiovascular disease and hyperlipidemia reinforced his risk.

Despite all of this, Tony was kind of like your everyman in that he didn't appear to be particularly unhealthy. He used to smoke a pack and a half per day, but that was 20 years ago, and he hadn't picked up the habit again. He drank moderately, mainly wine.

Tony's goals were to restore his health; reverse the effects of his stroke; lose the fat gained over the past couple of decades; get back into the gym; and show up his army buddies at their summer reunion in 6 months.

Risk Markers

TESTS	LOW	HIGH	TONY'S NUMBERS
Cardiac c-Reactive Protein (c-CRP)	0	1	**1.1↑ ***
Vitamin D	<30	>80	**17↓ ***

* = abnormal, out of range

HUMAN GROWTH HORMONE AND IGF-1. Human growth hormone is not a steroid hormone, though it is frequently referred to as one. It is a protein hormone, made up of amino acids produced by the brain's pituitary gland to spur growth. Typically, HGH is most abundant during childhood and adolescence, which makes sense because that is when our bodies are growing. In adults, HGH exists at lower circulating levels, though it continues to help maintain the health of organs, tissues, muscles, and bone. In all of us, there is a leveling off of HGH followed by a gradual decline that begins in the thirties and forties, though it is not as predictable as the decline in testosterone. Because HGH is also released mainly during sleep, if you're not logging enough hours with your pillow, your levels may be affected. Similarly, resistance training helps free up receptors so that HGH can bind at these sites; therefore, a lack of exercise can also lower HGH. Stress may have a negative effect on HGH production as well.

In the mid-1990s, the *New England Journal of Medicine* published a study by Daniel Rudman, MD, that showed that by administering HGH as a treatment, it is possible to reverse lean muscle decline, reduce fat accumulation around the trunk, and increase bone density in men in their sixties. Because HGH helps build lean muscle and bone, combining HGH with testosterone treatment can produce synergistic results for cardiac muscle and more. I prescribe HGH less frequently than testosterone, and HGH levels generally improve in the men I start on testosterone therapy, though likely the uptick of growth hormone is due more to effective physical activity and better sleep. I also recommend supplements, including amino acids like arginine, citrulline, and ornithine, that naturally stimulate release of HGH (more on this in Chapter 8).

Conversely, significantly elevated HGH is commonly associated with, acromegaly in adults (progressive enlargement of hands, feet, and hands), and gigantism (abnormally large size) in children. Abnormally high HGH is rare, however.

Related to HGH is insulin-like growth factor (IGF-1), also called somatomedin C, which is produced in the liver upon the release of HGH. It has growth-promoting effects on every cell in the body and also aids in DNA synthesis. IGF-1 deficiency results in short stature both for children and adults, and if severe enough, it requires supplementation. The research is somewhat divided on the role of IGF-1 in the aging process. Mutations that reduce IGF-1 have been shown to accelerate aging, and studies indicate that low levels of the hormone in humans may be detrimental in particular disease states. If a man's lab levels show that IGF-1 is persistently low, this is an indication of an HGH deficiency. I may consider writing a prescription for HGH. Both IGF-1 and HGH levels vary throughout the day. Stress, physical activity, nutrition, genetics, age, race, certain disease states, estrogen, body mass index, and endocrine disrupter chemicals may produce short-term or long-lasting fluctuations.

GETTING BETTER BLOOD WORK

By now, you're probably feeling overwhelmed. That's okay. I've introduced many new numbers to consider in the last two chapters.

There are many more unknowns than knowns with respect to hormones. Of course, that could be said for all the elements circulating in our blood. There are interactions between the amount you have of a particular hormone, where it travels to, what it binds to, how many receptors are present on the cell for it to link to, and finally what precipitates beyond that linkage. I don't fully understand this cascade of events, so I am presuming here a bit that by increasing hormone levels you're going to have better function. And the men I treat have the clinical responses to back up this assumption. For most hormones, the optimal level seems to be in the middle or high range, the upper 30 percent, without overdoing it. The exceptions are cortisol and insulin—these will serve you better if they're at the low end of the range, in the lower 25 percent, rather than in the middle or high range. Beginning with the next chapter, I will show you how making changes to your lifestyle combined with taking the right customized blend of supplements (Chapter 8) and cutting-edge interventions (Chapter 9). I can help you get your own hormones back to that sweet spot.

It really is all about balance, and I don't have the perfect formula for every person. Think about the seesaw analogy I used in reference to TSH, T3, and T4. Now think about all the different factors in your life, elements of your family history in addition to your biomarkers being weights of various sizes on either side. It's often difficult to get the seesaw balanced just right, so that it's parallel to the ground. That's what I'm aiming for, though—that individual equilibrium. It's a combination of factors so personal that it may even be different in identical twins. In Chapter 2, I stressed that you need to know yourself, and the tests I've introduced in these last two chapters will help you monitor your progress with your own stats.

Whenever I get into a discussion with people who aren't physicians or scientists about all the information I have presented here, I get similar reactions. *Wow, why aren't these things included in standard tests? So all I have to do is ask my doctor for these tests and I'm good to go?* Not necessarily. Some labs may offer "direct to consumer" services depending on state regulations—check with your local labs. In many cases, though, a doctor would have to provide a prescription for the tests. And, you'll want to make sure you have a trained medical professional lined up to interpret the results and provide wisdom and insight—to help you put together the pieces.

Recognize, too, there may be other obstacles to getting these blood tests done. Here are a few to consider.

OBSTACLE 1: YOUR DOCTOR. There are countless reasons your doctor may believe these types of blood tests are not effective or necessary. Your doctor may be conservative. He may even think that tinkering with your metabolism and hormones, especially testosterone, may be harmful. Such was the case with my patient Karl C.:

> I had been seeing an endocrinologist as my primary care physician for at least 15 years—the same individual, who was a very conservative endocrinologist. He would send me for a test or send me out to a specialist really at the drop of a hat to make sure that everything was in good and right order. I would normally see him

twice a year for physicals, and the relationship was a good one. I was in fairly good health, though one of the reasons why I'm part of Dr. Comite's program today is that I'm fighting my genetics. I have diabetes very deep in my family on both sides. I have heart disease that runs in my family on both sides. I need to be proactive or I'm going to wind up in an early grave.

With my primary care doctor, I felt like I wasn't getting enough. I wasn't healthy enough. I really wanted to do more on the preventive side, more than the general advice of "eat well, don't smoke, don't drink too much, and go to bed early." I wanted to go beyond that. So that's when I was introduced to Dr. Comite's practice, and I loved the science of it. That's what I was taken by. I loved the numbers. I like measurement benchmarking and really treating in a preventive way, as the practice does.

I'm sure I'm a typical client. It starts a little slow, and then it picks up. Everything since I've been a patient has gone in the right direction. Everything has gotten better.

Initially, I kept my relationship with my primary care doctor because, on occasion, you might get the sniffles. You might need an antibiotic, although fortunately, for me, that's relatively rare. I was very up front and honest with my doctor and said: "Here's my med table. Here's what I'm taking and here's why." He is a very pensive, thoughtful practitioner, so he took a look at it and asked me some questions about why I was doing this. I explained it to him. I put him in contact with Dr. Comite.

The next time I went back, he said: "I really don't like this. I don't like anything to do with this. I think you're being taken both intellectually and financially, and I think you should stop doing this." He said: "In the end, it's your decision, but as your primary care doctor, I'm strongly suggesting that you stop doing it."

To which I said: "Okay, I'll take it under advisement," and off I went.

I came back for the next appointment, and he said: "How are we doing?" I said I had decided to continue with Dr. Comite. He said: "Well, I've discussed this with my partners, and they agree with me. If you are going to continue to see Dr. Comite and you're going to continue with her program, then I can no longer be your doctor. You have a decision to make: Take me or take her. But I'm not going to be a party to this. There is no science behind it. There are no long-term studies. This falls under the category of 'nothing good can come from this.' This is similar to some of the early recommendations that women pursue hormone therapy. Later we found out that it was doing more harm than good."* He said: "Make your choice."

I made my choice. If he said he didn't want to see me, I didn't want to force him to see me because I'm not going to get the care that I need or want. So I walked away. What's unfortunate is that I had a great relationship with him. I think he genuinely liked me as a human being. He followed what I did professionally. I just think he was genuinely convinced that I was doing bad things to my body. He didn't want me to do that, and if I wasn't going to take his advice, then he couldn't be my doctor anymore.

—**KARL C.,** age 48, CEO of a financial institution

*Brief aside: This is not true for women in general and has been shown to be limited in many ways. Many articles support hormones for women as well. I'll discuss some of these in Chapter 9.

When Karl came for his first in-office visit, I gave him a jump drive with relevant articles—drawing from both the scientific literature and the popular press—that provided justification for the tests I was running. These sources also helped to give further insight into the particular conditions Karl was concerned about. I do this for all my patients. Karl tried to pass along the information to his doctor, but he didn't want to read it. Sometimes we don't want to know what we don't know.

OBSTACLE 2: TIME. Most internists typically see 20 to 40 patients a day. The average patient spends 8 to 16 minutes with his doctor annually. There are practical, medical, and economic factors at work here: It takes time to see each patient. We're not paying doctors for the time it takes to meaningfully confront the multifactorial issues a patient is facing. The main exception is when someone becomes a diagnostic enigma (think: *House*). So medicine remains predominantly disease based: *What brought you in, and how do we solve it?* There's a lack of incentive to focus on prevention and education about healthy lifestyle practices and treatment options. Patients won't get covered by their insurance, and doctors won't get paid. The best bet for starting a conversation may be to begin a dialogue at your annual physical. Schedule a follow-up appointment, and not just a phone conversation, to discuss your lab results. Think about what you want to know, come up with questions based on your results, and be sure the doctor can spend the 10 to 15 minutes that are needed to adequately discuss a topic.

OBSTACLE 3: INSURANCE COMPANIES. Health insurers are society's favorite punching bag for many reasons. The fact is, insuring people is a money-making enterprise, and companies structure their business so they can grow it. Therefore, some of these blood tests won't be covered, let alone standardized. Insurance companies don't want to uncover more disease, which would only lead to a need for more resources (e.g., physician's time, pharmaceuticals). On the contrary, these companies aim to insure a society that tests "normal" and "looks healthy." They have a limited vision. They focus on top-line issues and hope there is little or no negative impact on the quarterly reports for shareholders.

Insurers may raise objections, citing one or more of the following reasons. You should be aware of their possible protests.

- **Overtesting.** Too many tests make you a drain on the health care system.

- **Unnecessary testing.** Testing that's unwarranted causes too much harm and outweighs the good. Particular tests, based on what certain medical authorities advise, are deemed by insurers to be a waste of money. The other issue they will consider is what kind of trauma the test puts you through. Extensive or invasive testing may be done to search for explanations for any abnormalities found in your blood work.

- **Fishing expedition.** Casting a broad net and reeling in findings may yield no results. The investigation could be futile. For example, in the past, a sensitive CT scan of the lungs, when first available to patients, may have yielded an abnormal-looking lesion or a pulmonary nodule. Such a finding would necessitate a biopsy and then repeat testing several months later. With experience, interpretation is more finessed and definitive, offering tremendous value to you if it picks up an early lung cancer, for example. The argument suggests, however, that the patient goes through too much, with no promise of a definitive diagnosis, when a sophisticated workup is recommended using new technology and tools. Meanwhile, the additional testing costs more money.

Some people ask, "Wouldn't it be cheaper for health insurers to cover preventive measures now than to have to pay for more expensive health catastrophes later?" Not necessarily. Until rather recently, 2009 to be exact, hemoglobin A1c was not measured until someone developed diabetes. Now it's becoming a standardized test, though it's still not always used. Testing for hemoglobin A1c is likely to reveal thousands more individuals with diabetes, and, as a result, insurers may have to cover treatment for more patients, which increases their costs and decreases revenues. So this kind of comprehensive, in-depth testing is discouraged. The hope is that by the time there's real trouble, the patient will be over 65 or will already have a new health insurance policy through a different company. (It becomes like a hot potato, similar to those high-risk mortgages.) Why should insurance companies pay now for an impending disease when a diagnosis may be a few years down the line yet? At that later date, it will be someone else's headache.

OBSTACLE 4: MONEY. If necessary, are you willing to pay for these tests yourself? How much money are we talking about? It varies depending on how much is covered by your insurance, which laboratory is used, the types of tests, and whether your doctor thinks there are good reasons for the tests based on your health or even family history. Check that your physician will meet with you to authorize and review your test results.

You might offer to pay whatever amount is not covered by insurance for the follow-up appointment.

Using the stock market analogy, obtaining these tests is the same as getting insider information. Well, this insider info will impact your quality of life, potentially for years. Why wouldn't you want that?

> Once you start looking at all these reasons, you come back to: What's a good investment? What's a bad investment? People might spend $100,000 on a car. If you look at it from that standpoint, what difference will that investment make if you're dead? My partner, 63 years old, was worth $250 million and died of a heart attack. Do you think somebody would have caught his heart problems for 20 grand a year? But he just wouldn't see a doctor. He kept saying, "I'm better than that." Okay—you're better than that until you're dead.
>
> **—JOE NICOLLA,** age 55, business owner

The important thing now is that you take a step back and look at your puzzle as a whole. What do you see? Your personal history, family history, lifestyle, and lab values all interconnect, yet the pieces might not be fitting together quite right—a Rubik's Cube that you haven't figured out yet. Going forward, the place where you have the most control is in changing elements of your lifestyle. And while you may not believe it, these changes could lower your risk for diseases that run in your family or reverse damage that you've done to your body earlier in life. In the following chapters, I'll be addressing different aspects of lifestyle—sleep and stress, sex, nutrition, and exercise—and giving you practical information on how to optimize your health within these categories.

CHAPTER 5

THE SLEEP AND STRESS CONNECTION

Quality sleep is essential for healthy longevity. Reducing stress contributes greatly to well-being—and better sleep

You've got your personal health metrics. You've had your tests. Now how do you put it all together? Over the next few chapters, you will learn how to position your body in the sweet spot to optimize your health span. Your sex life will be revived, your diet will help you regain lost energy, and your exercise will become more efficient. With the right supplements and hormone therapy, you will support those efforts to slow and even reverse the aging process.

But your first stop is not the gym or the kitchen. The place to start making changes is in your bed. And I'm not talking about sex. At least not yet.

Stress and sleep are inextricably intertwined with each other and with your health. When you don't sleep well, you become stressed, and when you're stressed, you don't sleep well. You may be worried about work or your family, with thoughts that keep you tossing and turning all night. That results in poor-quality sleep, and you're exhausted in the morning, which contributes to stress at work. And the cycle begins again. This isn't just psychological—the levels of your stress hormone, cortisol, play a major role in determining the quality of your sleep and how long you stay asleep. Because all your physiological systems are interconnected, if you can't get adequate sleep and your stress is high, the efforts you make in eating well, exercising regularly, and taking nutritional supplements may not yield maximum results. When you're exhausted and stressed, it's hard to find the motivation to do anything but remain in survival mode. And this means you'll make expedient decisions but not necessarily the best ones.

Many clinical studies have shown that you need 7 to 9 hours of sleep in order for your body to repair itself. The combination of quality sleep and lower stress will actually help you be healthier.

QUALITY SLEEP: THE BASICS

William C. Dement, MD, the father of sleep medicine, who founded the very first sleep disorders clinic at Stanford University in 1970, defines sleep using two criteria.

1. A break between the conscious mind and the outside world. Even if your eyes stay open, being asleep means there's a sort of sensory wall that blocks your perceptions of your surroundings.
2. Something that is immediately reversible. For instance, in the presence of a loud, persistent noise, like your alarm, you will wake up.

Two other but no less important features of sleep are that it occurs naturally and periodically each day.

It used to be that the sun dictated your waking hours; you got up when it was light, and you slept when it was dark. It was a simpler time. Of course, you had to worry about attacks from four-legged predators and aggressive humans. Still, sometimes burning the midnight oil to finish off a big project seems equally as daunting or deadly.

Sleep requirements vary between individuals. A sleep cycle is around 90 minutes in duration, and during that time you go through each stage of sleep, with stage 2 (of five stages) predominating. You dream (stage 5) the most during the second half of sleep, and this is when you engage in rapid eye movement (REM) sleep. If you miss out on REM because you're not sleeping enough, there's such a thing as REM rebound that happens when you do finally get rest. In REM rebound, you'll get more REM than normal. I hear our patients report frequent dreams as their sleep improves.

Your body is primed to sleep, and from the moment you wake up, your sleep debt begins to build. This is the homeostatic component of sleep; it's always increasing throughout the day until you once again get some shut-eye. Imagine hiking uphill. By the end of that hike, you're going to feel fatigued. This is what happens to you every day with regard to sleep; it's that proverbial uphill battle. In addition to stress and other more pleasant environmental cues (like talking) that keep you awake, what also offsets this homeostatic component is your own biological clock. At certain times throughout the day, you get renewed bursts of energy, usually around dinnertime. On the other hand, your attention wanes and you lose your ability to stay awake in the early morning, in the early afternoon, and again at 1:00 to 3:00 a.m.

Your body's circadian rhythm, which governs sleeping, waking, and the appropriate production of hormones, is dependent on light cues and the time of day. Typically, your body temperature rises in the late afternoon, and as it begins to decline, you start to feel tired. Similarly, there is another rise in temperature in the early morning, around 5 a.m. At that time, your body is preparing itself for waking by releasing cortisol.

Nightcaps and Knockouts

Why alcohol and sleeping pills aren't the answer to insomnia

That late-evening drink you hope will put you out actually can undermine your sleep quality. Alcohol is a sleep interrupter and keeps most people from getting the deeper restorative sleep they need in the second half of the sleep cycle. Sleep after alcohol will often be fragmented, and you may wake up several times. The end result: You're more tired the next day. Even a cocktail as many as 6 hours before bedtime can disturb the second half of a night's sleep.

But that happy hour cocktail helps me unwind! That's what you're thinking. And maybe, for some of you, that happy hour cocktail turns into three or four or more. Sleep, stress, and substance abuse are linked in a sort of chicken-or-egg relationship. Did too much stress or lack of sleep push somebody to drink? Or did excessive drinking cause sleep disturbances and contribute to stress? After a while, it can become tough to tell what's the cause and what's the effect. The main issue is that the behavioral pattern isn't a good one.

Change patterns slowly. Cut back your alcohol intake by a quarter and then by a half. Or perhaps start off by drinking one glass of water for every glass of alcohol you consume. This helps you stay more hydrated. If you consume one or two glasses of wine each night with dinner, and then abruptly stop drinking, you may notice that your sleep becomes even more fragmented than when you are drinking. You may have more anxiety and nightmares. Give it time. Things will calm down.

Sleeping pills are no panacea either. A number of studies have shown that drugs like zolpidem (Ambien) and eszopiclone (Lunesta) offer no real improvements in sleep quality although a meta-analysis of Z-drugs showed that they did reduce the time it takes to fall asleep as compared to people who took a placebo. In a National Institutes of Health analysis, people got only 11 to 13 more minutes of sleep using a sleeping pill, and the quality of their sleep was just as bad as without medication. The short-term memory loss associated with taking a sleeping pill made them forget their tossing and turning, so they thought they slept better than they did.

Sleep is vital to a healthy body, so I do recommend sleeping pills or anti-anxiety medications if less intrusive methods are ineffective. It is important to address the issues that may be driving the sleep disorder, as well as undergo diagnostic assessments to rule out apnea. My typical guidance is to use sleep aids only if you absolutely need them. Melatonin, meditation, restorative exercises, therapy, and other approaches should be explored.

Our biological clock is a powerful modulator of behavior. In fact, Roger Smith, a researcher with the Stanford University Sleep Disorders Clinic, showed that it affects professional sports in unexpected ways. He studied the NFL and Monday Night Football and found West Coast teams who played Monday night games (beginning around 6 p.m.) in their own time zones (PST) had a 27.0 percentage point lead over East Coast teams. The reason being is that the East Coast teams were playing from 9:00 p.m. to 12:00 a.m. (EST), which is when body temperature drops and tiredness sets in. Other possibilities for West Coast teams' superior performance over East Coast teams included "home-field advantage" and that teams like the 49ers played closer to the time of day they train. Still, the evidence for the effect of circadian rhythm on athletic performance is compelling, and you don't need to be a pro athlete to apply these same principles to your life and schedule.

What's more, people can throw off their circadian rhythm with artificial light and their work habits. Bright light administered at night will disrupt your circadian rhythms so that you fall asleep later and rise later. This is why I recommend you keep electronics out of the bedroom and power down phones and computers at least an hour before bedtime to avoid the artificial light they emit. It's tough, and I'm guilty of failing to do so more than once a week. In fact, there's now a phenomenon known as *social jet lag*—essentially your social schedules are clashing with your biological clock, enticing you to stay up later and making you press the snooze button way past the 5-more-minutes mark. Conversely, light therapy is commonly used as a way to reset sleep clocks, especially for shift workers or individuals who travel frequently between time zones. Bright light administered in the early morning will help you get to sleep earlier and rise earlier. Supplemental melatonin in the evening or vigorous exercise in the morning can also help you to readjust your circadian rhythm.

GET THE SLEEP YOU NEED

America is now so sleep deprived that, according to the *Wall Street Journal,* fatigue-management consultants work with law enforcement groups,

Super Bowl–winning teams, and more than half of the current Fortune 500 companies on ways to maintain a consistently high-performing workforce and prevent accidents. At least 90 percent of my patients get less than sufficient amounts of sleep, and lack of energy is the number one complaint I hear, sleep deprivation obviously contributing. Being busy and sleeping less is in vogue, so much so that it's almost like a competition to see who can do the most while running on so little. You're taught to expect no less of yourself. "I can't, I'm tired" is no excuse.

Fact is, however, most people need 7 to 9 hours of sleep each night. You may need slightly more or less sleep than the recommended 8 hours, and you can tell if you're not getting enough by looking for these symptoms: irritability, moodiness, impaired memory, delayed reaction time, and slower reflexes. Sleep debt is very real, it accumulates, and it has consequences. One fewer hour of sleep per day means you'll carry that debt into the next day. If you've scrimped on sleep for an entire week, your sleep drive is going to be a formidable opponent during your 2:00 p.m. Friday meeting, when you experience a natural dip in alertness due to your circadian rhythm, or, more disconcerting and dangerous, during your drive home. Sleeping in for 12 hours from Saturday night to Sunday is often not enough. It takes much longer, up to several days, in fact, to get your sleep schedule back on track.

Did you know that prolonged lack of sleep makes you more susceptible to the common cold? Your immune system is more active during sleep, keeping you healthier when you get sufficient rest. Your health, mental acuity, libido, creativity, and memory all depend on sufficient sleep and keeping stress under control. Sleep trumps all in your path to healthy longevity.

The natural rhythm of sleep and wakefulness is determined by the cycle of hormones that are released by the brain. Change your natural sleeping patterns, and you change the secretion of cortisol and testosterone, as well as hormones that control appetite and metabolism. Increased or high cortisol, whether from stress or sleep deprivation, is a major factor in poor carbohydrate metabolism, leading to the development of insulin resistance and diabetes.

For instance, blood sugar and insulin are greatly impacted with chronic sleep loss, even after you've paid off your sleep debt. Sleep deprivation can age you more rapidly and may contribute to your developing diabetes if you are at risk. In fact, insulin response decreases with even just four nights of sleep deprivation (4 hours per night), and studies have shown that the response is similar to that experienced by diabetics and those who are obese.

Hormones that regulate appetite, too, are profoundly affected by sleep loss. Ever notice that you can't get enough of hamburgers and french fries during weeks when you don't sleep enough? The lack of sleep especially increases your craving for carbohydrates, and the increase in cortisol also makes you feel hungrier than usual. Sleep deprivation reduces the production of leptin (a hormone that tells your brain you are full) and increases production of ghrelin (a hormone that tells your body you are hungry). So if you sleep less than is needed several nights in a row, your body may feel as though it's been starved during that time. If leptin declines and ghrelin shoots up as a result of sleep deprivation, you may find it hard to keep from devouring the closest bag of chips or tub of ice cream.

Poor sleep and cortisol overload are a recipe for packing on the pounds, not just from eating too much but also because you will begin to store fat around your midsection. Many studies have noted that as average sleep time has decreased—from 8½ hours per night to 6½ hours per night over the last 50 years—average weight has gone up. So simply adjusting your sleep from 5 hours to 7 hours per night may actually help you lose weight.

If you don't get enough sleep, this can impact your body's ability to repair itself. Insulin-like growth factor 1 (IGF-1) and human growth hormone (HGH) are also secreted during sleep after the first round of slow-wave sleep and help promote cell growth and tissue repair. But if your cortisol levels are high, your body's insulin receptors will become occupied with insulin rather than be free to bind with IGF-1. Moreover, as you age, your percentage of slow-wave sleep declines noticeably. It's not yet understood whether age dictates this lack of deep sleep, or whether the lack of deep sleep contributes to the disorders of aging. Likely it's a combination. Studies have suggested that the activation of genes in the liver related to carbohydrate metabolism and growth hormone may be suppressed with inadequate sleep, again implicating the necessity of our night's rest.

Sleep deprivation can also interrupt the production of TSH (thyroid-stimulating hormone), reducing the amount needed at night to make sure your thyroid hormones are within range in the morning. Hormones, such as progesterone, and neurotransmitters, such as dopamine, tryptophan, and serotonin, have a role in brain function, sleep, and mood. These all shift with age and disorders of aging.

What's more, if you are stressing out at night about what went on during the day, you're going to have a tough time sleeping. Under calm circumstances, the pituitary in the brain issues orders to lower cortisol levels an hour before bedtime so that you can go to sleep. Yet when you're anxious, cortisol can shoot up just when you need it to bottom out. According to one study, the drop in evening cortisol in sleep-deprived people is up to six times slower than it needs to be for a restful sleep.

SLEEP AND TESTOSTERONE

If you're not sleeping enough, chances are your testosterone levels are lower as a result. A study published in 2011 in the *Journal of the American Medical Association* showed that sleep deprivation was linked to a dramatic reduction in testosterone levels in healthy young men (the average age was 24). During the first part of the study, the men were allowed to sleep 10 hours per night. Then they were only allowed to rest 5 hours per night for eight consecutive nights. After just 1 week of sleep deprivation, the men's testosterone levels had dropped 10 to 15 percent. While the link between sleep and testosterone production in men, especially those over 30, warrants further research, you already know what declining levels of testosterone can do: They impact your bone strength, your heart, your energy, your libido, your muscle mass, and your sense of well-being and vitality.

There's even evidence that men with erectile dysfunction are suffering from interrupted sleep, often in the form of sleep apnea. If you're experiencing erectile dysfunction, you not only should have your heart checked but also should have your sleep studied. And if you're not feeling rested when you wake up in the morning, it's another indication that your sleep quality needs a closer look.

So here's a big question for you: How do you feel when you wake up? Refreshed or exhausted? I've heard so many men come into my office and tell me that they are getting enough sleep—6 to 8 hours regularly— yet they are reporting feelings of fatigue and sleepiness throughout the day. In some cases, they have a tough time staying awake during a meeting. Though snoring is not always indicative of sleep apnea, it's one of the most telltale signs.

SLEEP APNEA

Sven B.'s wife's had complained of his snoring ever since they were first married. For a time, she found the sound comforting. That's when he was thinner, and the volume was tolerable—it was like a little hum that reminded her that someone was there next to her throughout the night. Fast-forward 20 years—Sven is 60 pounds heavier and diabetic. His snoring became so loud that his kids complained of hearing it in their rooms at the opposite end of the hall. His wife had moved, pretty much permanently, into the living room. She couldn't take the noise, although Sven insisted it wasn't as bad as she claimed. If it was so loud, he'd say, wouldn't his snoring, his gasping for air, wake him up? What's more, Sven said he felt fine—a little tired in the afternoons, but who isn't?

In fact, Sven's inability to get enough air was waking him up many times throughout the night. His upper airway was closing off, preventing oxygen from getting to his brain and body. He had sleep apnea but was totally unaware of it until he had a sleep study done. And he didn't go to get one of those until after a trip to Vegas with business colleagues. He had shared a room with a work buddy. Sven's snoring was so loud that his friend booked a separate room on the second day and stayed there through the remainder of the conference. Sven began to wonder, *Maybe my wife wasn't trying to be difficult. Maybe I do have a real problem.*

Definitions of Apnea and Interpreting Sleep Study Results

Obstructive sleep apnea (OSA): Your body tries to take in air, but with your airway being obstructed as your soft palate collapses, your lung volume remains unchanged. This gap in breathing usually lasts between 20 and 30 seconds, though it can last a minute or longer. Eventually, your body is working so hard to breathe that this effort will overcome the blockage.

Central sleep apnea (CSA): This is a complete cessation of breathing. There is no effort on your part to try to take in air despite your airway blockage. Central sleep apnea is much less common than OSA, occurring in about 10 percent of patients who walk into a sleep center. It is even more dangerous than OSA because there is no attempt to breathe, and death is more likely as it lengthens.

Mixed apnea: This is a combination of a central apnea followed by an obstructive apnea. I recently diagnosed this condition in a physician who slept 8 hours every night yet still reported fatigue. Both he and his wife are doctors, yet it was not evident to them that he had obstructive and central sleep apnea, a life-threatening diagnosis.

Apnea: This is a complete cessation of breath lasting for at least 10 seconds.

Hypopnea: This is less severe than apnea, though it does disrupt your sleep and factors into your diagnosis.

The sleep specialists you see will calculate your apnea-hypopnea index (AHI). This is how the AHI breaks down.

- If your AHI greater than 5 but less than 15 events per hour, you have mild apnea.
- If your AHI is between 15 and 30 events per hour, you have moderate apnea.
- If your AHI is over 30 events per hour, you have severe apnea.

Sleep apnea is the partial or complete blockage of the upper respiratory airway during sleep, a condition that's more common in men than in women. Think about holding your breath underwater, except there's no pool. You're in your bedroom, which has plenty of oxygen, but you're not getting any air to your lungs. That's apnea—a cessation of breath that can last from 20 seconds to more than a minute. If you tried to hold your breath underwater for that long, you might be pumping your way to the surface fast. It's extremely detrimental to sleep quality, especially REM sleep. And if it goes unchecked and is severe enough, sleep apnea may result in death. Daytime sleepiness, mental fog, and snoring witnessed by a bed partner are the most frequent complaints that prompt folks to seek medical attention. Gasping for air during sleep is another symptom. Each time one of those gasps occurs, the brain "wakes up," and it pulls you out of whatever sleep stage you're in. As a result, your sleep is often shallow and fragmented. Cortisol also rises, as your body stresses itself trying to take in air and consistently failing time and again. Alcohol and certain antidepressants, sedatives, and hypnotics will make things worse.

The gold standard in diagnosing sleep apnea is an overnight polysomnography by an accredited sleep center. The night technician will lead you through the process in which electrodes are attached to your scalp, face, legs, arms, chest, and abdomen. Many people experience some trepidation when faced with an overnight sleep study. They are worried and feel uncomfortable out of their own bedroom. All this may prevent them from falling asleep or staying asleep, which can skew results. Because of these problems, I now use a home monitoring system called SleepImage.™ It's a lot simpler than a formal sleep study; you apply the two cardiopulmonary leads yourself and go to sleep in your own bed. The beauty of the SleepImage is that you can test your sleep on multiple nights. We can test somebody one night after taking sleeping pills and another night without; one night with alcohol, another without. The machine delivers a detailed report of your sleep, which is then scored by a technician. We evaluate the report and make recommendations. If sleep apnea is evident, then referral to a sleep center is in order to confirm and assess treatment options, such as continuous positive airway pressure or CPAP, commonly known as "the face mask."

Even if you have mild to moderate apnea, a doctor will likely want you to have an overnight study in which you'll be fitted with a face mask that uses continuous positive airway pressure. This device forces your upper airway to open during sleep so you get oxygen to your brain and body.

There are two types of CPAP devices—the nasal pillows and the full face mask, which covers your nose and mouth. The nasal pillows are inserted into your nostrils, similar to nose plugs; most sleep doctors and patients prefer these because they're less obtrusive. Still, a good sleep clinic will allow you to test both machines for comfort before you turn in for the night. No matter which you choose, however, the treatment mechanism is the same. A constant stream of pressurized air flows through the CPAP mask and forces open the airway, allowing for unobstructed breathing. It is a tough adjustment, but if you stick with using the CPAP device nightly, it can greatly improve your quality of life and allow your partner quality sleep too!

A final note: The drawback with managing sleep apnea is that you're using a mechanical device to fix the problem. It's treatment, certainly, though not a cure per se. In order to remain apnea free (or at least close to it), you have to be diligent about using the CPAP machine nightly and making sure it's titrated to the appropriate level to keep you breathing throughout the night. (Doctors will want to see your apnea-hypopnea index under 5 events per hour.) Other treatments for apnea, while less common, include dental procedures and devices, positional therapies, and bariatric surgery, like gastric bypass or gastric banding. Losing weight can make a real difference and, for some men, can greatly improve sleep quality. As you might have already predicted, cardiovascular disease, stroke, diabetes, high blood pressure, obesity, and neuromuscular issues such as restless leg syndrome tend to go hand in hand with apnea.

Sven B. arranged an overnight study at a sleep center, which diagnosed him as having moderate to severe apnea (AHI of 27 events per hour) and brought him back in for a CPAP study. When he was using the device, his snoring nearly disappeared, and he slept soundly.

THE ROLE OF MELATONIN

Melatonin is something that I commonly use to help my patients get to sleep. You've probably heard of it, and you may even have purchased it in supplement form at the drugstore. Released by the pineal gland, melatonin is sometimes referred to as the "Dracula of hormones" because it's typically released at night, sometime around 9 o'clock. It promotes sleepiness, and production continues for about 12 hours. Again, though, the brain is sensitive to light cues, even artificial light, so the pineal gland may not get the message to release melatonin if you're constantly bathed in light from fluorescent bulbs and electronics. What's more, research is inconclusive about whether it helps you increase your total amount of sleep.

I have two male patients who were sleeping little, and they also had very low testosterone levels. They were functioning, although exhausted all the time. After evaluating their lab results, in addition to their medical history, family history, and lifestyle, I started them on testosterone and several other medications and supplements, including melatonin. It took about 6 months, but when they came back, they said their ability to fall asleep and stay asleep had improved dramatically. As one of them told me, "Stop my testosterone, but don't dare take away my melatonin." What's more, even very low dosages, just 1 milligram per night, were effective, though that is not necessarily true for everyone.

Other supplements and medications can be useful to help regulate sleep. These will be discussed in later chapters.

THE STRESS CONNECTION

Not getting enough sleep has massive health implications, and stress can set off a whole host of other problems. Too often I see men deny or simply rationalize being overwhelmed; even if they admit to feeling too busy or fatigued, they don't realize the impact stress may have on their health. Many just consider that constant stress is acceptable, the norm, the way life is lived.

While the absence of stress is seldom noticed, its presence can bring about a host of ailments or even awaken symptoms that have been lying dormant, accumulating over time. Some diseases and signs or symptoms that are affected by stress include heart disease, bacterial and viral infections, shortened telomeres (damaged DNA; see Chapter 12) and more rapid aging, autoimmune conditions such as rheumatoid arthritis and multiple sclerosis, arterial inflammation, impaired carbohydrate metabolism, and weight gain. What's worse, a compounded effect of any of these variables could increase your risk of serious illness. High levels of cortisol—which is secreted by the adrenal glands—lead to increased storage of body fat in the belly region. Appearance aside, this is the worst place for fat to reside. This visceral fat, which surrounds your vital organs, secretes a hormonelike chemical, or cytokine, called interleukin 6 that causes an inflammatory response. This is the same thing that happens with insulin when we overeat and can lead to diabetes, heart disease, or cancer. It can also result in metabolic syndrome, which is a cluster of symptoms like high blood sugar, poor cholesterol, hypertension, and excess fat, especially around the middle. It increases your cardiovascular risk. Typically men with metabolic syndrome tend to have even lower testosterone levels at a younger age than other men, in my clinical experience.

Stress can do serious harm, and the root of it may begin deep within your brain in the limbic system, which is a cluster of structures that control emotion, motivation, punishment, reward, and the expressive response to memory. Stress also can be more involuntary than that; your body's actions are governed by the autonomic nervous system (ANS). The ANS, if you recall from Psych 101, is made up of three components, all of which impact both your mental and your physical well-being.

You remember the fight-or-flight response that kicks in when your neighbor's angry bulldog tries to take a nip out of your calf? It engages the sympathetic nervous system. Heart rate goes up, digestion slows, and cortisol and norepinephrine levels rise as your body prepares to either dropkick that annoying furball with teeth or flee the scene. By the way, the body can react similarly to an intimidating boss or high-pressure board meeting.

Engaging the parasympathetic nervous system produces the opposite response. This is commonly referred to as the rest-and-digest state. The production of stress hormones slows, and your body gets back to leisurely activities like salivation, urination, defecation, sexual arousal, even creating tears. There's a third system, known as the enteric nervous system, which is associated with digestion. Neurons—more than 100 million of them—line our gut, from the esophagus to the anus. Research suggests that these neurons may also be responsible for those feelings of butterflies in your stomach, a feeling of stress.

If you're constantly frazzled and crazed, you're likely engaging the autonomic nervous system quite often. Add to that anxiety affliction with irritable bowel syndrome, and your enteric system may be telling you that you're also suffering from depression. Stress is difficult to quantify; however, it would be reflected in cortisol levels if you did a blood test. Morning levels may be between 6 and 10 or 8 and 12 micrograms per deciliter (mcg/dL). In the evenings, your cortisol level is usually 6 mcg/dL or under.

Stress triggers cortisol, which, in turn, affects your ability to metabolize carbohydrates and may contribute to prediabetes and diabetes by driving up your blood sugar, insulin, and hemoglobin A1c. High cortisol can affect your immune system, which is why you may find yourself fighting a cold soon after a stressful event, like the start of a new job or the death of a loved one. If you recall Noah N. (from Chapter 4), he had very high cortisol and was prediabetic, too. He was unable to keep off weight around his trunk.

Many people cannot just guess at their cortisol levels by how they feel. There isn't always a connection between feeling stressed out and physiological response. Alex B., who is a lead counsel at a major company, is a good example. His is a high-pressure job, especially when he is litigating in court, yet his cortisol registers only a 6 mcg/dL, which is at the low end of the reference range. Alex's body has a way of maintaining balance and control that causes his cortisol to remain in an acceptable range. Conversely, some people may claim to feel no stress, which may well be true, but if they have their cortisol measured, they discover it's high. It's pretty common for people living in New York City to have cortisol levels in the twenties and thirties. Another patient of mine saw his cortisol drop from 25 mcg/dL to 6 mcg/dL when he relocated from Battery Park in New York City to New Hampshire.

A common misconception is that the stress hormone is situation specific, rising—like blood pressure—in stressful situations and lowering when life calms down. Sure, that does happen, but more typically cortisol rises and falls with the ebb and flow of the day.

It is impossible to know what your cortisol is doing under the surface regardless of whether you claim to be stressed or not stressed, happy or disappointed with your life, frazzled or not. This is where Eastern medicine can help. It teaches that you don't want to have extreme reactions to either happiness or sadness. You want to be able to take everything in and process it in a balanced way, maintaining equanimity and clarity. This is a great thing to strive for, but it's difficult to achieve. Restorative exercise like meditation, yoga, qigong, and tai chi can help you reach that equilibrium while lowering cortisol, too.

Despite your best efforts, that balance may be impossible to achieve at times. One of the worst experiences I've had with managing stress was at a medical conference. It was 1994, and I was responsible for organizing a major conference at Yale University called Hearts and Minds. *New York Times* health writer Jane Brody was the keynote speaker, and hundreds of people were expected to attend. I worked day and night for weeks in preparation while trying to balance an already hectic professional and personal life, with two young boys at home. Within 24 hours before the conference, I learned that two key people who were supposed to help me introduce speakers and manage the program were unable to attend. I got only a couple of hours of sleep that night.

When I woke up, instead of feeling anxious and overwhelmed, I felt nothing. I had no trepidation, no butterflies in my stomach. I had nothing left. I was numb. Sure enough, a day later I came down with a severe upper respiratory infection. It was clear to me that I had worn myself down completely, so much so that my cortisol levels plummeted. I had no reserves left. (This was made all the more ironic because the connection between mind and body was the topic of the conference!) In the days leading up to the conference, I'm sure my cortisol was extremely high. I was constantly fighting to survive. It was fight or flight 24/7. As a result, the high level of cortisol sustained my body; cortisol is a steroidlike hormone, which can also suppress inflammation, fever, and acute signs or symptoms of an impending illness. Cortisol and steroids mask symptoms, but you can't sustain such high levels indefinitely, which is why as soon as the stress dissipated, I got sick.

There are many similar stories about people who get sick after doing something quite successfully. Your immune system is vulnerable to stress. Increased cortisol can make you more susceptible to the bugs going around your office or family and less able to shake an infection. When your immunity drops, your body is not in a strong position to resist disease, of any sort. Researchers at the Carnegie Mellon University demonstrated this when they injected study participants with a cold virus. Those participants who reported chronic stress for a month or longer were much more susceptible to getting sick than were those who reported only mild to moderate levels of stress. In upcoming chapters, I'll suggest some strategies and supplements that can help boost your immune system's functioning.

"THE GOOD LIFE" AND AGING

One of the most remarkable longitudinal studies ever conducted began in 1938 at Harvard University and continues today. Starting with 64 sophomores, the Grant Study of Adult Development grew to include a total of 268 men from the all-male Harvard classes of 1939 to 1944. The goal of the study was to observe these men over time to better understand the human condition—what makes humans happy, what makes us succeed, what leads us down the wrong path, and more. The observations were meticulous. The men received both physical and psychological examinations, and over the years study investigators checked in with them about their personal and professional lives. Harvard psychiatrist George Vaillant, MD, took over the research in 1961 (and has since written three books on the study participants). While nearly all the subjects were worried and anxious from ages 25 to 35, Dr. Vaillant explains that almost all of them became successful by age 45. By the fourth decade of life and onward, they felt that they had found their place in the world. Similarly, Gail Sheehy explains in her book *Passages* that the twenties and thirties are a stressful time characterized by self-discovery, growing up, and negotiations. Like Vaillant, Sheehy considers the forties and beyond to be particularly rich, and part of that comes with knowing yourself better. The good news for some of you, then, is that you're already in this sweet phase of your life, and some of the stress of uncertainty ought to be behind you. What's more, Vaillant says there's more to look forward to. Thirty percent of the Grant Study men have lived to be in their nineties (only 3 percent were expected to hit this milestone). The study showed that avoiding smoking and not abusing alcohol were the most important things one could do to live longer. Also, good marriages predicted longevity. And the key to happiness? Love.

STRATEGIES FOR REDUCING STRESS

Anything the body takes in can be perceived as a stressor, whether it's over-the-top great news or an October report telling you that the bottom just dropped out of your company's fiscal year budget. Although it is difficult to avoid stress in our fast-paced world, it is possible to manage it. The first step is to identify stressors. Your electronic devices may be a major source of stress and the easiest to control. With smartphones, especially the ones provided by your employer, people expect you to be at their disposal all the time: after hours, even on weekends. The tether between you and your phone(s) will feel like a short one, pulled tight. As an overextended overachiever, however, your productivity will likely suffer, and you'll be doing harm to yourself if you don't give your mind a break.

GIVE YOURSELF BOUNDARIES. Power down the phone. Don't just keep it on vibrate or silent, because guess what? Every time your phone lights up telling you there's a new message, your brain gets a little squirt of dopamine (a neurotransmitter that acts upon the reward and pleasure centers in the brain and is associated with novelty). Obsessively checking your phones—because, you never know, that next message may be great, and at the very least, it's new—can keep you craving that dopamine hit. It may also raise cortisol levels. If you can give yourself the space to truly disconnect, it will help lower your cortisol levels and give you a chance to come up for air.

SLEEP WELL. Keep a regular schedule, especially for going to bed and awakening, because it aids in reducing stress and creating metabolic and hormonal balance. If you are accustomed to staying up late, try going to bed 15 minutes earlier and see how you feel. Each week, go to bed another 15 minutes earlier until you are getting 7 or 8 hours and you can see the difference the extra sleep makes.

STEER CLEAR OF BLUE LIGHT. Late at night, your eyes and brain perceives the blue light from TVs, computers, tablets, and smartphones as daylight and signals you to begin the waking process just as you need to sleep. Trade your cell phone or laptop for a cup of warm tea and a relaxing read (not a thriller or a stock market report) on printed paper, not on a Kindle or an iPad. On weekends or vacation, turning off all your technological gadgets can lead to creativity, so be spontaneous and go on an adventure hands free!

GET SOME EXERCISE EVERY DAY. Light aerobic exercise, like walking, is one of the easiest ways to work off the effects of cortisol and reduce stress. Exercise is a positive type of stress that elicits an immune response, which requires a recovery period in order to rebuild your muscles. However, too much exercise can lead to symptoms of overtraining: fatigue, soreness, lack of appetite, lethargy, lack of motivation, illness, injury, decrease in performance, and irritability. So don't over train. Restorative exercise can be anything that makes you happy or that takes your mind off stressors: golfing with your buddies, taking a hike with friends, meditation, yoga, massage, tai chi, or simply exercising alone.

HYDRATE PROPERLY AND EAT WELL. Adequate hydration and nutritious food are needed to maintain balanced energy levels and make your day a smoother sail. After all, if there is no healthy you to do your job, then you won't be at work anyway. Eating and taking care of yourself is not selfish; it's your *right,* and it's a necessity.

GIVE YOUR EYES A REST. The amount of strain we put on our eyes daily leads to neurological fatigue in the optic nerve and brain. Be cognizant of how much strain you are putting on your eyes, and step away from the screen often enough.

REWARD GOOD BEHAVIOR, NOT STRESS. Have a delicious, not-so-good-for-you meal, an ice-cream cone, or an alcoholic beverage when you've had a good string of exercise and healthy eating, not when you're under increased pressure at work. After all, if you have too much to drink after a stressful day at work, your body knows no difference between the two stressors. Then you have to wake up and balance out your body before starting your day.

GO FISHING WITH A BUDDY; FIND SUPPORT. Support is also something men don't think about much; however, you can do a lot of good by surrounding yourself with people who *add* to the value of your day, not take away from it. Laughter is a great stress reducer; hang out with loved ones and friends who make you feel good. Put some wind in your sails instead of adding an anchor.

TAKE A 15-MINUTE VACATION. Sit in a quiet room, close your eyes, and clear your mind. Do this at least 15 minutes a day. It also helps to get away from your current routine on occasion by trying something new or going on a vacation. Even a weekend out of town or a day trip can do wonders for your psyche. Go on a long hike or bike ride. A 15-minute walk in the middle of your day can do wonders for your eyes and brain.

I'm my own worst enemy. That's the biggest challenge. Always has been. I have the tendency to slack off and drift with the familiar comfort of a low-grade depressive lethargy. I'm sure I inherited this trait. I'm a child of Holocaust survivors. My parents, both resistance fighters during the Nazi occupation of Holland, lost friends and family and were direct witnesses to the horrors. During my early to middle adult years, I lost two wives to cancer—one in 1981, the other in 1998. Both left me with young children. The specter of those events still haunts me. In the past, I found comfort in food and alcohol, even though I am aware that in doing so I am reinforcing negative habits. What motivates me this time around is working with a spiritual leader as a way to deal with the accompanying stress and lingering emotional issues. I move ahead knowing full well that I can live a healthy and fulfilling life as I enter the senior years—and that I can experience these things I don't want to miss, such as the following:

- Seeing my children and grandchildren grow up
- World travel
- Living and growing older alongside my wife (her family history is filled with 90-year-olds!)
- Finishing my novel, and perhaps experiencing another Red Sox World Series!

—SIG VAN RAAN, PHD, age 66, psychologist, consultant, and writer

Determine what you want your life to be like, and start setting goals. Start by looking at how you sleep, which affects how you live the amount of stress you're under. Whether or not you will make change depends on your attitude. If you are confident that change is possible, then it will be so. A good night's sleep will help free your mind, and you'll wake up feeling refreshed, strong, ready to live life to the fullest—and have better sex! Turn the page.

CHAPTER **6**

GREAT SEX, YOUR SECOND ACT

How to boost your libido, gain firmer erections, and make your sex life sizzle again

R emember the summer of fill-in-the-blank? You were in your twenties, strong, happy, feeling alive, and filled with a seemingly insatiable hunger for sex.

Then, you met a girl, settled down, and had kids. The sex five times a week turned into once or twice a week or less, maybe once a month. Now, 10 or 15 years later, you can't remember the last time you and your wife had sex. Living together has become more like being roommates. You and your wife are desperately seeking solutions, devising exit strategies, or even just existing together.

You may have another big problem, one that's always on your mind and causes anxiety which manifests itself in a particular kind of avoidance behavior. Perhaps you repeatedly tell your wife, "Not tonight."

There's a program you want to watch. You've brought home work from the office. Or you're going out to play poker with the boys.

You're embarrassed by the fact that sex is no longer a regular part of your life. It once was something you could count on to make you happy, to relieve stress, and to help you sleep better. You know your wife is frustrated too, but you can't talk to her about your difficulties in getting an erection. What if she felt you were less of a man? So you stay silent and continue to worry and avoid intimacy. You just don't feel in control of your life anymore.

The men who come into my office are at various stages of their intimate relationships. Some are in a supportive, loving marriage or partnership; others are facing real struggles. I see many who are recently separated or divorced, contemplating new partners or simply exploring options. What do they have in common? About half of them notice that their interest in sex is minimal, if that. In fact, that is sometimes the driving force behind their relationship issues. When I launched Women's Health at Yale in the early 1990s, I thought my female patients would complain most about their own loss of libido, especially how their poor body image impacted their desire for sex. I was surprised to learn that many of my female patients instead were worried about their husbands' diminishing sex drive and sexual function. Their men seemed to not miss the intimacy that was absent from their relationships. Not infrequently, the women would acquiesce and agonize privately without saying anything to their partners, for fear of making things worse. Viagra wasn't on the market yet, and there were no commercials touting the benefits of checking your testosterone or making your loved one feel loved.

Ironically, hormones in women hitting their forties are shifting toward a relatively more dominant androgenic pattern, causing an increase in sexual desire in most. Meanwhile, men of the same age are feeling the drop in testosterone. Their levels are not what they once were at age 18 or 25. What I hear from men is *When I want to make love, I can't get an erection. I can't maintain an erection the way I used to*. They don't have morning erections anymore, or maybe these occur only infrequently instead of daily as they once did. These men do realize that something is lacking, but they submit to the mystery of it all. They adapt to the incremental changes over months to years, and let it go at that.

How much sex men want differs, with couples reporting less activity than singles. There is a wide range in what men consider enough sexual activity—from multiple times a day, to once every other month. Even in their prime, some men are perfectly happy with once a week or month. What partners in steady, long-term relationships report most commonly, is having sex a couple of times a week.

Over the years, this may change. While some men do their best to compensate, making small adjustments here and there, libido becomes elusive. Other men may feel like the joy of life is waning. They may feel empty—their enthusiasm gone—and they start reexamining, questioning everything. Some men will channel their efforts in to other activities, like exercise. But if they don't experience an increase in muscle and stamina, their disappointment can lead to bewilderment, and even depression.

I would estimate that 30 to 50 percent of the men I see claim their interest in sex is much lower than what it once was. Yet they often explain it away: *What else can I expect after so many years? Isn't it natural to lose interest in sex?*

It just seemed to happen. I would have never said that I had any less of a desire for sex. I would look at a beautiful woman, and I would certainly think about it. Still, I wasn't seeking closeness and intimacy as often as I would have in the past. You kind of put it off, saying you're busy, and your life is pulled in different directions. Maybe it's part of what I might call a maturing issue. You don't really think of any specific physical portion. You just kind of accept it. You look in the mirror after you get to a certain age, and you think: Gee, there are a lot of wrinkles around my eyes. You don't really see them coming, and yet, they're there. So this was kind of the same thing. My desire for sex was diminished. I didn't feel it happening. I didn't even realize it was happening. I think that's why sometimes your eyesight goes bad so you can't see your wrinkles as you get older. Then you put your glasses on and go, "Whoa!"

—JOHN HORAN, age 57, general contractor

If I revisit our car analogy, when it comes to sex, the Kinsey Institute for Research in Sex, Gender, and Reproduction argues that the problem is with the engine. The inability to maintain an erection or reach orgasm is like when a car's "check engine" light comes on. The car is not going to run as well, but it's still going to work (at least for a while). The loss of desire or libido presents more of a challenge. In this case, it's like the engine won't turn over and the car won't start at all.

Such was the case for my patient Jason Rockwood. When he first came into the office, he was only 35 and had been noticing changes in his sexual drive and function since age 33. Jason had always prided himself on being a very sexual person, and he acutely felt this shift in his character. He felt as if his body transitioned from summer into winter in a span of 2 years. His sex life was not what it had once been. As a result, he sought help from numerous sources. In those 2 years before coming to see me, he had spoken with his primary care doctor and experimented with a variety of treatments such as Viagra, Cialis, and even Caverject, an erectile dysfunction (ED) drug that is injected directly into the penis. While these medicines worked—he said the Caverject gave him "porn-star erections"—he still didn't have the sexual desire to match his newly upgraded hardware.

The mechanical component behind less-than-desirable sexual function is just part of the equation. It is, however, the piece that has received the most play in the media. A study by the Congressional Budget Office showed that in 2008, pharmaceutical companies collectively spent more than $300 million on direct-to-consumer marketing of ED

Your Sex Preferences

Asking yourself a battery of questions about your sex life—and answering honestly—can help you evaluate your desire and preferences and compare them with how you felt 10 or 20 years ago. This little exercise can be helpful in adjusting your course back to sexual vigor and satisfaction.

- What was your best sexual experience? How long ago was it?
- How often do you think about sex?
- How often do you want sex? How often do you actually have sex?
- Do you have dreams about sex? Who is the partner in the dream?
- Do you achieve orgasms? How do you feel after an orgasm: relaxed, elated, or drained?
- Does sex occur most frequently after you drink?
- If you're in a long-term relationship, who initiates sex more often, you or your partner, or is it about equal?
- Do you and your partner both feel sexually satisfied after intercourse?
- Is penetration your favorite sexual activity?
- Do you enjoy foreplay?
- Does your partner seem satisfied with your sexual relationship?
- Do you wish you were more open-minded about sexual activities?
- Do you feel comfortable talking to your partner about new activities you would like to try?

There are no right or wrong answers to these questions. Compare your answers with how you felt at the age of 25. These insights will show how you've changed as a sexual being and provide ideas for achieving greater sexual satisfaction.

drugs, surpassing statins, sleep aids, and antidepressants. This statistic indicates just how hungry men are for ways to improve their sexual function.

According to the Massachusetts Male Aging Study, an estimated 18 million to 30 million men are affected by ED. Erectile function refers to a host of actions: achieving an erection, having a hard enough erection for penetration, and maintaining an erection for yourself and your partner's pleasure. Men may experience difficulty with one, some, or all of these. Premature ejaculation may also surface at different times, though less frequently in older men than in young men. More commonly, however, men have mentioned they are troubled by how little ejaculate they're producing and the diminished forcefulness of their ejaculations.

These stories and countless others are proof that erectile dysfunction is often a complex problem, one that's rarely purely physical. It follows, then, that medications offer only a temporary fix. The little blue Viagra pill may help you right now, and taking Cialis will even give you that boost for up to a day and a half, should you be in the mood. Still, there are underlying hormonal and psychological pieces to the low-libido and erection concerns that warrant further attention.

The hormonal shift and declining interest in sex may start happening for men as they head into their forties. If you recall from Chapter 1, testosterone begins declining annually by 1 to 3 percent in men around early to midthirties. Not surprisingly, the change in hormone levels coincides with so-called midlife transitions, possibly initiating the crises that are so common. The brain is not firing in the way it used to. It is no surprise that all the men introduced in Chapter 3 were impacted by testosterone levels that were less than adequate.

Low testosterone may be one of the underlying problems if you're having trouble with the following:

- Decrease in number of morning erections

- Lack of interest in sex

- Losing desire shortly after engaging in foreplay

- Losing your erection shortly after penetration

- Trying to get through quickly before losing your erection and/or desire

- Losing your erection and/or desire before your partner can become aroused
- Lack of forcefulness in ejaculation
- Lack of intensity in orgasm
- Decrease in semen

Low testosterone isn't always something men can immediately perceive. In fact, some men may not even notice particular sexual issues. They recognize changes in other parts of their lives, and once they address their hormone levels with treatment, they realize just how much their sexual function has been impacted. My patient Alan S. had this kind of experience.

A 150-mile bike trip Alan took with his son convinced him that his body wasn't working as it once had. He got through the first day well enough. Although he cycled all 75 miles the second day, his pace was slow, his joints hurt, and he couldn't keep up with his son and the other riders. Soon thereafter, we reconnected at a high school reunion. During his first office visit, we discussed his sexual function. He told me that he hadn't noticed a decline in his libido, except for the fact that he was going through a divorce and therefore wasn't having regular sex. After reviewing Alan's blood work, however, I found that his total and free testosterone levels were low. Once his hormone levels were optimized, he began working out regularly with a trainer. He soon entered into a new relationship and noticed the difference in his sex life.

Having low testosterone doesn't necessarily equate to having ED or experiencing a decrease in libido. By the same token, having testosterone that's on the higher end of the optimal range doesn't guarantee a stellar sex life. I've seen plenty of men with higher than average T who have no libido and iffy performance. It isn't just the number attached to the testosterone level; it is also about the relationship between the brain's signals, your interpretation and feeling, and your penis. This connection is neither direct nor simple.

If you begin to notice a change in erectile function, you may be worried it will happen again. If you perceive your libido isn't as strong, you may grow frustrated or embarrassed. When your mind or body is grappling with stressors, your sympathetic nervous system— the one that produces that fight-or-flight response—will be in overdrive. That's great when an angry dog is nipping at your heels, but not good when you're about to have sex. While the sympathetic nervous system is active during sex in order to reach climax and ejaculation, the parasympathetic nervous system first needs to be engaged for you to become aroused. Everything has an impact on this delicate mind-body connection. It's not performance on command. Some men may prefer to dissociate sex from feelings, yet when the act becomes a challenge, there's an emotional aspect that can be quite profound. One of my patients, Wade B., described the feeling as "soul destroying"; it was as if his inability to function sexually was undermining his very being.

Having never had erectile dysfunction before, I had no real understanding of what it felt like. I'm in a long-term relationship with my girlfriend, but this happened during the early stages. I felt paranoid about how she reacted. I remember having this sense of: Why would a woman want to be with someone who couldn't perform in this way? All of the fear that's associated with losing someone you love comes flooding in because there's a notion that if you can't perform well sexually, the relationship cannot be sustained; sexual performance is too significant a part. That's the big thing—the fear that I'm not going to be the person she is going to want to be with.

For me, there's something that's almost indescribable about being a functioning, virile, powerful man that gets undermined when you have that experience. It seems like the entire ego and personality go as flaccid as the penis. Emotionally, it's really difficult. It was challenging at first—explaining it and understanding it. There's a secondary fear of: Is this going to stay this way? Is it going to get worse? I know from reading, for a lot of people with ED, there's a huge psychological component.

—WADE B., age 63, CEO

Alcohol (which dilates your blood vessels, then constricts them), recreational drugs, smoking, stress, anxiety, and lack of sleep are all contributing lifestyle factors of ED. Smokers, in particular, have almost twice the risk of ED as nonsmokers, and men who smoke and have arterial sclerosis are even more vulnerable. Often obesity also affects sexual function. Fat tissue is rich with aromatase, which, as mentioned in Chapter 4, is an enzyme that converts testosterone into estrogen. Estrogen will prevent testosterone from working the way it should. And, as testosterone levels fall, fat increases and lean muscle declines. Illness and other health conditions—whether chronic, like diabetes, metabolic syndrome, and high blood pressure or acute, like an upper respiratory infection—often have an effect on sexual function. When your body is focused on healing, sex is not a number one priority.

In some cases, ED may actually serve as a warning sign, heralding the onset of a more serious disease. If you have a problem with cholesterol, plaque, and inflammation, it's likely to obstruct these thin pudendal arteries before the coronary arteries. If there's a vascular obstruction around the penis preventing the bloodflow necessary to achieve erection, chances are there are also other blockages in your system. Erectile dysfunction is a strong predictor of heart attack, stroke, and death from cardiovascular disease. This doesn't mean that every man with ED will have heart disease or that every man with heart disease will have ED, but the connection is strong. In fact, the researchers of one study recommended that every man with ED be evaluated for cardiovascular disease.

Other disorders like a weak heart that can't pump blood adequately may lead to insufficient filling of the penis's vessels. If that's the case, you may be able to get an erection, but it may not be a particularly strong one. High blood pressure may be another contributing cardiovascular factor. Not unlike radiator hoses that become hard and crack with age, the arteries can become stiff, less responsive, and more resistant to allowing blood to flow freely. High blood pressure may also cause some resistance within the corpus cavernosum, the chamber in the penis that fills with blood in order to achieve erection.

Inflammation within the arteries and sluggish bloodflow (remember all those sugarcoated red blood cells) are common in individuals with diabetes. It follows that the arteries of the penis may also be affected. The dysfunction occurs in the endothelium, the cells that line the inside of the blood vessels. Diabetes not only affects the vessels themselves, but also may impact nerve tissue and sensations in the skin. As a result, you might not enjoy sexual contact as much as you did in the past. Evidence shows that good blood sugar control can minimize these risks. Still other conditions that may cause ED include atherosclerosis (hardening of the arteries), kidney disease, and multiple sclerosis.

TALKING ABOUT SEXUAL FUNCTION: A CULTURAL TABOO

Men have great difficulty talking about their frustration with sexual function. Wade, Alan, and John never shared their fears with anyone other than their partners and my team. It's not an issue that they talked about with any sort of regularity.

Today, the dialogue about sexual function and andropause is growing, but it's still a very hush-hush topic. The commercials that target men with andropause and erectile dysfunction use expressions like "stepping out of the shadows" or "don't be afraid to bring up these concerns with your doctor, it's just a number." A similar dialogue about menopause occurred decades ago. Women didn't want to talk about the change. They were afraid they'd be perceived as "old" or as useless members of society. They wanted to remain physically attractive and worried that not being able to conceive made them less desirable. Eventually, though, as women rapidly advanced in the workplace and started families later in life, the stigma of menopause began to disappear, though it's still evident. The acceptance of andropause may follow a different trajectory, but eventually it will be recognized as a legitimate issue that can't always be solved with Viagra. Hormone optimization, which I touched upon briefly in Chapter 4 and will return to in Chapter 9, is the future.

> It was frustrating, to know that you have a problem that no one will acknowledge as a problem. It's kind of like depression when people will say: "Oh, it's all in your head." With andropause, there's a shame and insecurity around the topic, when there really doesn't need to be. It's not a personal defect. It's a chemical defect. When you get the chemicals adjusted, the defect goes away, just like with depression. Much like mental illness, we don't openly speak about hormones and hormone therapy. I feel like hormone therapy is where treating depression was 30 years ago.
> —**JASON ROCKWOOD,** age 35, marketing executive

GREATER LIBIDO, STRONGER ERECTIONS

The official diagnosis for erectile dysfunction is this: Erections that are too brief or not firm enough for sexual intercourse 75 percent of the time. Men are concerned before they reach this point, however.

There are many options for retrieving sexual function. You've no doubt seen the commercials, and the part about calling a doctor "in the rare event an erection lasts more than 4 hours" is so ubiquitous, it's become a punch line in pop culture. All of this makes it hard to believe that sildenafil (Viagra) has only been on the market for a little over 10 years. Other oral ED drugs are even newer to the public. This class of drugs also includes tadalafil (Cialis), vardenafil (Levitra) and vardenafil (Staxyn), and avanafil (Stendra), all of which work by improving bloodflow to the penis during arousal. They're typically taken 30 to 60 minutes before sexual activity and, in general, should not be used more than once a day. There are exceptions for some of my patients with severe erectile dysfunction. They are on daily Cialis and also take Viagra to augment erections as needed. Cialis can be taken up to 36 hours before sexual activity or can be used daily at a lower dose. Injections administered directly into the penis, like alprostadil (Caverject), work by widening the blood vessels, causing the penis to become engorged with blood. Another option is inserting a medicated pellet (Muse; alprostadil) into the urethra; the pellet can trigger an erection within 10 minutes. To try out any of these medications, you will first have to see your doctor to be cleared for safety and receive a prescription. Several supplements, like fenugreek extract and L-arginine, which will be discussed in Chapter 8, also increase bloodflow and improve erections. Your lab data is a good place to start to ascertain your particular needs. Your doctor can help you interpret those numbers in relation to your subjective experiences and medical history.

Using medications or supplements to improve your erectile functioning is dependent, in part, on having adequate testosterone levels. At the first signs of flagging interest or difficulty maintaining an erection, the little blue pill (or others like it) can have a huge impact. After a while, however, it may not do the same job. It's typically low testosterone, not necessarily the body's desensitization to the drug, that leads to this diminished function.

Once I address the low testosterone either through treatment with testosterone itself or through treatment with human chorionic gonadotropin (hCG) to trigger release of testosterone (see Chapter 9), you may find that the common ED drugs work much better. Using these treatments in combination, you can regain the same healthy performance that you had in years past.

A few weeks after my patient John Horan began injecting hCG twice weekly, he was chasing his wife around like they were newlyweds all over again. By upping his testosterone levels, he was also able to put on lean muscle and lose some weight, dropping two pants sizes in less than 6 months. He was overcome by a general feeling of wellness that he never realized he had lost. He said it was like an "aphrodisiac."

Alan T. felt similarly. *Sexy* was the word he used. Testosterone was helping to improve his sex life and his physique, and both made him feel more attractive. His partner saw the difference, and friends did too.

Jason Rockwood, whom I started on hCG, enjoyed the desire he once again felt—that longing to be close to someone. He called it "amorousness."

It's like I gained a couple of years back. I'm finding myself kissing in a way that I haven't kissed in years. One of my lovers said, "You're so frisky. I haven't seen you this frisky before." That's such a silly word, but it's an important word because it really sums up how I'm feeling. I'm happy again, and I'm interested again, and there's a kind of energy again that had just been gone for the last couple of years. To see that come back and to find your body reacting to things in the way that it used to—it isn't something new, it's just that it's something I used to have and lost. I'm getting that back. Viagra makes it possible to have sex even when you're not in the mood, but the cool thing about hCG is that it put me in the mood again. All the time, really. And I loved that.

It's bizarre, but analogies about autumn and spring—they're real. I've literally felt a seasonal transition in my body. It's like when dead trees come back alive in the spring and you start to see the leaves budding. It's a subtle, almost invisible process, but over the course of the month, it's very obviously not winter anymore. That's what it feels like. It's funny. Going through it, these analogies do come to your mind about fire and ice and hot and cold and summer and winter. You realize how much your body is a product of these kinds of natural rhythms, and that if you can adjust these natural rhythms, then you can live in a perpetual spring.

—JASON ROCKWOOD

FEELING LIKE A COLLEGE KID DURING SPRING BREAK

When the sexual desire returns, it can be overwhelming. I've had patients call me asking me to dial it back a bit—they couldn't think about anything but sex, and it was taking over their lives. Sometimes, their partners aren't fully prepared for the uptick in libido. After I started John Horan on hCG, his wife, Karen, was wary. She was going through menopause and underwent a hysterectomy at 43; she wasn't always in the mood. Within weeks, John was waking her up in the morning looking to have sex before work, and she was running the other way. In time, she saw how good John was feeling, and she, too, became a patient of mine so that she could focus on her own hormonal health. She hopes that she and John can get back on the same page sexually, given that their level of sexual desire had been fairly equal throughout their marriage.

Even though you may have the libido you had in your twenties, thanks to testosterone, you might not be able to perform like you did in college. Your refractory period—the time between ejaculation and the ability to achieve another erection—probably won't change back to what it was when you were having sex three or four times in a night. Wade noticed that his sexual function improved immensely after being treated with testosterone injections and Cialis. Still, he was frustrated he couldn't make love quite as often as he wanted. Roughly 10 times a week seemed to be his maximum, even if he wanted more. Alan hasn't noticed any performance issues, though he insists on having sex with his girlfriend every night. One evening, she asked him why he was so concerned with making sex a daily occurrence. Was it a kind of competition? Was it because he could? When he thought about it, he decided it was the latter. He didn't know if at an older age it would be possible to get an erection every day. For him, there was still a fear about age and the undeniable limitations it may pose.

WHAT IF HORMONES AND ED DRUGS DON'T WORK?

Sometimes there are mechanical issues that no hormone therapy or little blue pill can remedy. One patient of mine had tried numerous treatments for ED, and nothing appeared to be working. While his health and libido improved dramatically on my program, sometimes his erections weren't fully satisfying. After he went to a specialist, I discovered that there was leakage from the vessels that fill the penis, making it physically impossible for him to maintain an erection. It was like trying to fill a bathtub without a stopper. I had to find a way for his chambers to fill artificially. Now he uses a surgically implanted device that helps him get an erection when he wants one, for as long as he wants it. Another option is a malleable implant, which bolsters erections with surgically implanted rods.

Vacuum devices for ED, also called pumps, offer an alternative to medication. The penis is placed inside a cylinder, and then the pump draws air out of the cylinder, creating a partial vacuum. This causes the penis to fill with blood, leading to an erection. An elastic band worn around the base of the penis maintains the erection during intercourse.

If ED is caused by a blockage in an artery leading to the penis, surgery can often restore bloodflow. Good candidates for this surgery are typically younger men whose blockage stems from an injury to the crotch or pelvis. The procedure is not recommended for older men with significant narrowing of the arteries.

When there's blockage in an artery of the heart, inserting a stent sometimes can help keep the vessels open. There is an experimental procedure for doing the same for the arteries leading to the penis if cholesterol blockages are interfering with erectile function (a condition known as arteriogenic erectile dysfunction). Urologist Irwin Goldstein, MD, invented the technique, and a recent investigation of 30 men who had undergone the surgery showed no major adverse events after 30 days. Meanwhile, the stents helped improve bloodflow to the penis, and intercourse success rates rose.

The majority of men who suffer from ED, however, will not require surgery. Some men blame their partner for their problems. They may be in a relationship that's 20, 30, or 40 years long. The ad hominem attacks pile up. Someone's fat, someone's a cheater, someone's a liar. In a different scenario, the discontent is more quiet and cerebral. No one is really talking about the fact that sex is absent from the relationship, and each party may be inwardly blaming the other. In these situations, communication is often the best place to start in terms of treatment. Even if ED, low testosterone, or physical appearance becomes an issue, psychotherapy can be beneficial. A therapist can teach you and your partner techniques to improve intimacy. Therapy can also help couples adjust to the use of vacuum devices and implants.

It's natural to feel angry or embarrassed when dealing with sexual function and desire. But don't forget that your partner is also affected. Talking openly about it will help reassure your partner that you haven't lost interest.

If sexual function becomes a hurdle and you worry about your performance, you can take steps to lessen your anxiety. One of the ways is to shift the focus from genital stimulation to pleasuring in other ways. You take turns—you focus on pleasuring your partner, and then your partner focuses on pleasuring you. Eventually you can progress to genital stimulation, with intercourse still being off the table. It helps to see that there are other ways to reach orgasm besides sexual intercourse.

We are taught so little about sex during our youth and young adulthood that we all stumble and struggle into our own imperfect translation of our sexual experiences. If sexuality is a continuing education, a lot of us are scrambling to make up course credits. In a realm that's clouded by ego, myth, and advertising that preys on anxieties, getting the facts about sex can be difficult. It's individual, and there are no guidelines that work for everyone. Only the things that work for you will be useful and, ultimately, applicable. The more you do to keep yourself at your healthiest, the more likely you will be able to enjoy pleasurable sexual interactions.

CHAPTER 7

BUILDING A HIGH-PERFORMANCE BODY

Follow a natural diet of high-quality macro- and micronutrients and a strategic fitness plan designed to combat muscle loss

In 2008, I was overweight and sluggish, and I decided to get back into shape. Everyone reaches that point where they feel like crap; then they look in the mirror and say, "I look like crap, too." Well, I had enough crap! People told me, "John, you're just getting older, it is what it is." That wasn't acceptable to me. There had to be a better way.

Test results came back: I had the classic high cholesterol, high triglycerides. You can find that out by going to any doctor. But Dr. Comite focused on other markers that no one else looked at: my hormone levels, testosterone, growth hormone levels, homocysteine. All of them are factors that affect your health and how you age.

She gave me a full nutrition and fitness plan, and I stick to it (with the occasional cookie). I started to feel better and could work out harder. Within a few months, I dropped weight and my energy shot up. My weight loss, 15 pounds, isn't the big thing. My body fat percentage dropped considerably, which means I replaced a lot of fat with muscle. The spare tire around my gut is gone. I have far more energy and feel like I have taken back the things that had slipped away when I wasn't taking care of myself.

Here's the best part: I'm part of a weekly soccer game, what we call the Old Timers Soccer Club, and my performance from before I started with Dr. Comite to now is night and day. You can't even compare.

—JOHN BELLIZZI, age 55, vice president, global head of business development

Food is your fuel. If you don't properly fill your body with the right kind of nutrients, you won't feel healthy and energetic, you won't lose weight, and you won't build muscle. It really is that simple.

What complicates things for just about everyone is how food is manufactured and sold. Most of the food you buy is loaded with the stuff that makes it taste incredibly delicious and encourages you to keep eating: sugar, fat, and salt.

Convenience is another lure that leads you down the path to a poor diet. You're overworked, overscheduled, and prone to making poor choices. On every corner, there's a fast-food restaurant or a convenience store full of packaged, processed foods. The ease of access to quick food makes it difficult to say no and even more difficult to spend the time making healthier meals at home. Unfortunately, those convenience foods are often nutritionally poor and calorie-dense. So, here we are, with two-thirds of the country overweight or obese.

Why do we eat? We need to sustain our body's energy demands, not simply to satisfy our hunger. Signals within our body get miscommunicated or changed as our cells turn over. Maybe, in the times of hunting and gathering, satisfying hunger was equivalent to meeting energy demands. We were underfed and undernourished. The difference now is that we are overfed, and still undernourished.

It wasn't so long ago that our relationship with food was quite different. Go back a few hundred years. We all participated in finding food, and our bodies were good at processing what was available to us—mainly lean protein and vegetables. When we did come upon, say an apple tree with apples that were ripe, we would eat all we could. As such, our bodies became adept at storing carbohydrates because they were rare in comparison to other foods.

There's something more insidious about today's continuous overload of sugar than simple weight gain. If sugar stays in your bloodstream too long or sugar levels spike too high, insulin can't work fast enough to clear the sugar from your body, and the excess glucose becomes corrosive to your tissues. That's why the body needs to use carbohydrates immediately or convert and store them as fat—so sugar doesn't cause tissue damage. Type 2 diabetes happens over time at the cellular level. Blood sugar spikes if you eat successive carbohydrate-heavy meals, raising insulin levels continually higher, causing insulin resistance. Contrary to popular belief, insulin resistance is a process, and it doesn't happen suddenly.

This damage was triggered decades earlier. Insulin resistance is a condition known as prediabetes. This is when the insulin that is circulating in the blood remains high even when you are fasting. Unfortunately, the insulin has lost its ability to store and clean up the circulating sugar in your system. If this situation continues over years, the pancreas will eventually burn out and insulin production stops. (This is what you typically see in an individual with type 2 diabetes.) Now you are a diabetic, and unless your body is provided with insulin, it will be unable to clear sugar from your bloodstream.

Poor food choices, overeating, and inadequate physical activity—along with your hormone levels and genetic makeup—conspire to increase the odds of poor sugar metabolism. Type 2 diabetes typically emerges in older adults. In fact, it was formerly called adult-onset diabetes. Now we're seeing this form of diabetes being diagnosed in children as young as age 5. Type 2 diabetes differs from type 1; typically, type 1 diabetics are more likely to be born with the inability to produce insulin and other hormones that control carbohydrate metabolism.

But I'm not prediabetic or diabetic, you say. *Why should I be concerned about sugar?* Here's something that may be of interest to you: When insulin is present in the bloodstream, you do not burn body fat. You're in fat-storage mode. Yet when you prevent blood sugar and insulin spikes during the day by eating intelligently, at regular intervals, you allow your body to burn fat throughout the day. Bottom line, you want to avoid insulin or sugar spikes because they may cause weight gain and contribute to you becoming a diabetic.

HOW TO AVOID SPIKES IN INSULIN TO PREVENT WEIGHT GAIN AND DIABETES

Eating at intervals of every 3 to 4 hours keeps your blood sugar stable and helps you avoid the cravings that might send you in search of high-carbohydrate snacks. Eating intelligently means choosing foods that keep you feeling full and satisfied. This is why a high-protein diet is so effective at helping people lose weight. Protein tells your body not to store energy as fat but to burn the fat stores that it already has. The result: You lose fat; you lose weight.

MOVE TOWARD HIGH PROTEIN, LOW CARB. Protein is a muscle builder, and it should always be an important part of your diet, especially as you age. You've read about what naturally happens to your body as you get older: Testosterone drops and you lose muscle, regardless of whether you're a triathlete or a couch potato. Muscle helps you metabolize sugar, and so less muscle means the body loses the ability to metabolize carbs as well as it did when you were younger. See the cycle? This can lead to insulin resistance, weight gain, and an uptick in cholesterol and triglyceride levels. The downward cycle begins.

Enter protein. Consuming lean protein—such as fish or fowl or a portion of meat a little larger than the size of your palm (not the Big Texan on the steak house menu)—for some meals has multiple benefits. Vegetables, legumes, certain grains, and dairy sources are also good vegetarian options that will give you similar positive results. First, protein signals satiety, so it helps you feel full and stop eating at the right time. Protein also takes longer to digest than carbs, so you feel fuller longer, and lowers glycemic load, as discussed on pages 145 to 146. Additionally, protein provides the raw material needed to repair your daily tissue damage, not just your muscles after a workout. For example, your body replaces blood cells every 100 days or so. That's a lot of cell turnover, and almost every system in your body is constantly renewing itself. When you work out and break down muscle, protein is essential to fuel the repair. Many of my patients have learned that they need to eat more protein to sustain the lean muscle that develops as their workouts improve.

Eating protein throughout the day also helps you burn more calories because it takes more energy to metabolize protein than carbs (sugar) or fat. We call that the *thermogenic* effect of food. By limiting simple carbohydrates (cookies, cake) and slightly increasing protein intake you can burn your fat energy stores. Remember, though, not to overdo it. The body can't process more than approximately 35 grams of protein in one sitting. That's about a 6-ounce steak. Any excess protein you eat per sitting will be stored as fat, which defeats the purpose of eating more protein and fewer carbs.

So, exactly how much protein should you eat? A moderately active individual (exercising 30 to 60 minutes three to five times per week) may require 1.2 to 1.4 grams of protein per kilogram of body weight. To calculate your weight in kilograms, divide your weight in pounds by 2.2. If you weigh 170 pounds, it is equivalent to 77 kilograms. Now multiply 77 by 1.2 or 1.4, which is approximately 92 to 108 grams of protein intake daily. Remember, it is best to go slow in making changes. Focus on implementing these dietary improvements over the course of a month or two—not in a day or a single week. Protein metabolism can be hard on the kidneys, so drinking extra water will help your body adjust.

One of the easiest ways to increase quality protein in your diet is by eating a true breakfast. Having an all-carb breakfast of a muffin and banana is no good for you. Get in the habit of fueling up with a protein-based morning meal. Also, eat within 30 to 60 minutes of waking to break the fast you experienced during sleep and to signal the body to start burning energy. Some good choices for your morning:

- Greek yogurt with 12 to 15 grams of protein

- Cottage cheese and berries

- A protein shake with at least 25 grams of protein combined with fresh or frozen berries

- Almond butter on whole wheat toast or on a banana

- Two or three free-range eggs mixed with vegetables

- Last night's chicken and asparagus leftovers

- Steel-cut oatmeal with protein powder, flavored with cinnamon

When I make recommendations to patients, starting each day with a protein-rich breakfast is at the top of the list. It sets you up right. If you continue to get protein throughout your day, eat at regular intervals, and watch your carb intake, you'll be on your way to a healthier you—and weight loss, if that's your goal. Additionally, I encourage my patients to try extra tips on the following pages.

MAKE SURE YOU ARE WELL HYDRATED. Ninety to 96 ounces of water a day are needed for optimal body function. Few of us drink that much. As you increase your protein intake, it is even more crucial to hydrate. Here's a suggestion: Drink two glasses when you rise in the morning and one or two with every meal and snack. Also, keep a water bottle at your desk. If you feel sleepy or hungry during the afternoon, it could be that you are feeling the effects of dehydration. Drink water until your urine is light straw yellow. I recommend you drink as much water as half your weight in ounces per day, especially if you're working out. For example, if you're 180 pounds, you should be drinking 90 ounces or $2\frac{2}{3}$ liters of plain water daily. Metabolism requires a lot of water. You can lose 20 ounces of water or more in an hour of exercise. If you're even slightly dehydrated, your metabolism slows, undermining the other changes you've been making to optimize fat burn and muscle gain. Try to limit water close to bedtime, however, as you don't want to interrupt your sleep for bathroom runs.

ADD PROTEIN EASILY WITH SHAKES. Protein shakes are a fast, convenient way to boost your daily protein consumption and satisfy that empty feeling between meals. They're especially good before or after workouts. (Research shows before is better.) Whey protein isolate powders are available in any health food store in various flavors. Check to be sure there are minimal added ingredients. Keep it pure. Whey can be very beneficial for vegetarians who need additional protein without additional calories. If you are a strict vegan, try supplementing with pea or rice protein powders.

FILL UP ON FIBER. Fiber, like protein and fat, helps you feel full, takes longer to digest, and slows the absorption of sugar into the bloodstream. It also helps maintain digestive health and lower cholesterol. The daily recommendation is around 25 grams of fiber. Eating lots of vegetables will help you get there. Other high-fiber foods are apples, beans, and nuts. Grains like oatmeal (steel-cut is best) and quinoa are also good.

AVOID ALCOHOL. Cutting back or completely eliminating alcohol is one of the most effective ways to lose weight and improve your blood sugar levels. Think about it: Beer has one of the highest glycemic values of any beverage—a double shot of sugar from alcohol plus carbs. Wine, too, is very high in carbohydrates. Having one or two glasses of wine a couple of nights a week is generally not a problem, yet you may need to modify your habits once you understand your personal health metrics. For example, one of my patients loved his two to three glasses of red wine nightly and did not want to give up alcohol. No matter how well Sam P. did in every other area—his nutrition, his workouts—the wine contributed to his diabetic status, partly because of his metabolic profile. Once he decided to cut down and finally stop drinking wine altogether, his carbohydrate metabolism was excellent. This process did not happen overnight—it took a couple of years for him to move in that direction. When I asked whether it was challenging to go without the wine, Sam chuckled and said, "Not at all. I like the way I feel and don't miss the wine." He was able to do more at work and play harder. He felt stronger. Most important, diabetes is no longer his inevitable destiny.

KEEP AN EYE ON THE INDEX. I'm talking about the glycemic index (GI), one of the best tools for combating diabetes (and losing weight). This measure indicates how a typical serving of a certain food will raise your blood sugar. The GI scale ranges from 0 to 100. I recommend that patients pick foods with low glycemic indices, or those with GIs less than 45. The higher a food's glycemic index, the quicker the food is absorbed into the body and the higher it raises your blood sugar. Consuming smaller amounts of higher glycemic foods less often is another way to balance. You don't have to cut out your favorites altogether. In season, I'll eat pineapple and mango, which I love, yet stick mostly to berries and apples because they have a lower GI. Find the healthier versions of foods you like and make them your go-to choice.

Glycemic load (GL), on the other hand, refers to the amount of insulin that is released to process the sugar. In most cases, the higher the glycemic index, the higher the glycemic load. By pairing a carb with a fibrous or protein-containing food, however, you can reduce the glycemic load of the meal or snack. Be careful of eating too much of any low GI food since this will affect the GL. Pasta is a good example; it is tricky. Certain pasta can have the same GI as carrots. Yet unlike carrots, consuming less than ½ cup of pasta (typically suggested serving size) is not likely (just think about how much pasta you pile on your plate!). Higher amounts of pasta will drive up the GL even though the GI is still relatively low. Another way to look at it is that fiber- and protein-containing foods generally are lower glycemic and will offset and lower the rise in blood sugar and insulin that carbohydrates produce. Find a GI and GL app for your smartphone. You can also visit KeepItUpTheBook.com for more information on the glycemic index and glycemic load.

AVOID CARBS AT BEDTIME. Sleep is an important part of your day—it's when your body does most self-restoration. Crucial to this process are human growth hormone (HGH) and insulin growth factor (IGF-1), typically produced at night. IGF-1 is triggered by the presence of HGH and is released by the liver and skeletal muscles to help build and repair tissues. It's crucial that you give your body the chance to do this as efficiently as possible. Recall from earlier chapters that IGF-1 shares the same receptor sites as insulin. When insulin is present because you've indulged in a high-carb snack before bed, IGF-1 is pushed aside. Eating carbohydrates at night hampers this recovery process because insulin levels increase, preventing IGF-1 from binding to receptor sites. Remember from Chapter 5 that alcohol interrupts sleep and contains carbs on top of that.

If you have a sweet snack like cake or cookies or even a low-glycemic fruit like strawberries or a pear right before bed, you inhibit your body's recovery and restoration process. But there's a way to skirt the problem: If you're hungry, combine berries with Greek yogurt or nibble on a handful of nuts. And when you eat enough protein, good fats, and fiber throughout the day, you'll be less likely to feel compelled to nosh on sweets at night. That's the effect of emphasizing protein, eating a balanced breakfast, and hydrating properly.

SKIP THE JUICER. Turning fruits into juice is a surefire way to get a dose of concentrated sugar and drive up your risk of diabetes. Better to grab one orange and eat the whole segments (including membrane) than squeeze a few citrus fruit for the juice. You need the fiber from the whole fruit; the juice alone is almost as bad as plain sugar. Remember to combine your fruit with protein. One exception would be veggie juice, because it is likely to contain far less sugar than fruit.

EAT ALKALINE FOODS. Foods have either an acidic or alkaline effect on the body as they're digested. An acidic profile causes inflammation and is not good for our bones—think of a tooth dropped into a can of Coke; the tooth dissolves. What are the best highly alkaline foods? Easy. Vegetables. Any food that's naturally grown and vibrant in color is good. Each day, try to eat as many colors of the rainbow as possible. Salads make it easy.

Take my patient Wayne Hickory, for example. He switched to a vegetable-based diet, noticing that it was getting a lot of attention from news outlets and medical experts claiming a daily intake rich in greens reduces cardiovascular disease. In genetic testing, Wayne had a single-nucleotide polymorphism (SNP) identified as 9p21, putting him at greater risk for having a heart attack (see more about this in Chapter 10). Research has shown, however, that if you eat a diet high in raw fruits and vegetables, you can essentially reverse this risk to zero. The vegetarian path was looking like a smart choice, though Wayne also wanted to make sure his diet was balanced. If you're a vegetarian, you can ensure you're not depriving your body of that essential protein it needs by eating tofu, legumes, dairy, quinoa, rice protein, and spirulina. Those are some staples, yet often I find that in order to get enough protein, physically active vegetarians would end up eating too many calories, too much food in terms of bulk, or both. So they take a protein supplement. Wayne does. (See Chapter 8.)

BALANCE OMEGA-3S AND OMEGA-6S TO REDUCE INFLAMMATION. By now you may be aware of the many cardioprotective benefits of omega-3 fatty acids. You find these in oily fish like salmon (not smoked), tuna, cod, halibut, and herring. Seeds, nuts, and avocado are other good sources. Walnuts are highest in omega-3-fatty acids, followed by almonds, cashews, pistachios, and Brazil nuts. Omega-6s are healthy, natural fatty acids found in most vegetable oils, chicken, and beef. Your body needs omega-6 fatty acids for proper neural function, but you don't want to overconsume them, either. Omega-6s are considered pro-inflammatory, while omega-3s are thought to be anti-inflammatory. If you lack omega-3s and are heavy on the omega-6s, you promote inflammation and raise your heart disease risk.

Eating a typical American diet, you may be getting too many omega-6s and not enough omega-3s, the ratio being about 30 to 1, respectively. The more desirable proportion would be about 4–6 to 1 to reduce your risk of inflammation, which is the primary driving force to disease and aging. The "good" omegas fight inflammation in the body, which is one of the biggest enemies of long-term health. Remember my discussion of cardiac C-reactive protein (c-CRP) and homocysteine in Chapter 3? Both are inflammatory markers, and the lower your number, the better. Omega-3s can help reduce your c-CRP and homocysteine, keeping your arteries wide open.

If you have high cholesterol, particularly a high LDL, along with a nutrient deficiency such as a lack of B vitamins, you would be well served to increase your intake of omega-3s.

SNACK CREATIVELY. Snacks should follow the same high-protein to low-carb ratio as your meals, though on a smaller scale. Use your imagination with combinations. Some ideas: sliced apple and a handful of walnuts; Greek yogurt with berries; apple with a teaspoon or two of nut butter (cashew, almond, or walnut butter is a better choice than peanut); pear with a piece of cheese about the size of two dice; a hard-cooked egg; cottage cheese and low-glycemic fruit such as an apple or peach. When possible, select fruit such as berries, or an apple, a pear, or a kiwifruit, which have lower glycemic indexes than fruits such as pineapple, mango, and watermelon. Refer to the glycemic index list at KeepItUpTheBook.com.

A lot of our patients struggle with timing their meals. Remember Phillip B. from Chapter 3? He travels a lot for work and pleasure. Or consider Dave M., who is so busy caring for his ailing father that he often forgets to eat regularly throughout the day. If this always-on-the-go lifestyle sounds similar to your own, you may want to plan ahead.

Prepare healthy snacks on Sunday before the start of the workweek. Make things quick and easy—Greek yogurt, apple slices and almond butter, a protein shake.

SUBSTITUTE SPICE FOR CALORIES. This is an effective strategy for controlling calories. Instead of adding syrup or honey to sweeten your steel-cut oatmeal, add cinnamon (sometimes referred to as the poor man's insulin because the spice helps to lower blood sugar) and some chopped apple or berries. Instead of ketchup, mayo, or barbecue sauce, go for lower-cal grainy mustards, plain horseradish, or garlic. Instead of high-sodium hot sauce, try crushed red pepper. You have an entire spice rack to utilize. The goal: Get the most flavor for the least caloric impact.

REWARD GOOD BEHAVIOR. Give yourself an "attaboy" treat. For example, did you eat breakfast every day and hit five weekly exercise sessions? If so, reward yourself with one treat during the weekend.

PLAN AHEAD FOR SUCCESS. If you fill your day with a handful of good food choices, you'll automatically push out the bad ones because you'll be too full to eat the food that isn't healthy for you. Over time, you'll feel so much better that you won't want to indulge in junk. Flip to the Appendix where you can follow the Precision Health Questionnaire. It will help you to track your meals and get an accurate sense of what you're eating and how your body is reacting to it. (For additional questions, visit KeepItUpTheBook.com.) Numerous studies have shown that people who keep a record of their diet—even when they don't count calories—become more cognizant of their food intake and ultimately lose weight.

Now that your body is fueled properly, the next step to optimizing your metabolism is fitness. No matter where you are on the fitness scale—whether sedentary or highly active, or somewhere in between—engaging in the right types of exercise is a crucial step in getting on track to your optimal health. As we shared in Chapter 2, the best fitness routine for you will be determined based on your personal health metrics. Your lab tests, your family history, your own past medical history, and other lifestyle choices will all be relevant as you move forward.

MAKE A MUSCLE, AND MORE

I work out every day. It used to be drudgery. It's easy now. I love my workouts. If I don't do them every day, it's depressing. I mesh weight training and cardio—high reps, one set to another. I'll knock out 1,000 reps in 45 minutes. My girlfriend says I'm crazy. A 40-year-old client of mine is a physician who designed the workout. He said I wouldn't be able to do all of it for 3 years. I mastered it after a few months. When I play sports with other people in my age group now, I'm way beyond them.

—**DICK DEFLURI,** age 62, founder, Abundance Wealth Counselors

I see male patients at all levels of fitness, from ultracompetitive athletes to those who haven't moved with purpose in decades and everybody in between. This is what I share with them: "No matter what you've done in the past, to leverage your gains in the areas of sleep, stress, sex, nutrition, and supplementation, exercise is essential." Following the food tips listed previously is like filling your sports car with the best grade of gasoline. Omitting exercise is like keeping your car parked in the driveway. Perhaps you do move from time to time, though you don't stay on a regular schedule. In that case, your "car" will show wear. Just as your tires may lose air, your windshield wiper blades may grow dull, and the brakes may lose their responsiveness, your body will "rust," susceptible to disorders of aging like obesity or cardiovascular disease.

For the athletes in my practice, keeping up their fitness routine isn't a problem. Exercise is already a part of their day. Yet there is still more for them to do: tweaks to make, new things to try, balance to attain. For everyone else, including beginners and even folks in the middle, making time for exercise in their weekly schedule can be challenging. Prior commitments, between work and family, or frequent travel pose hurdles. But know that constant excuses will not allow for positive outcomes, and your stats are unlikely to improve much. Commit to an exercise plan, start out slow, and stick to it. Beginners and on-again, off-again exercisers may wonder how to jump-start. The best place to begin is with a grasp of what it means to be physically fit.

THE KEY COMPONENTS OF A FIT BODY

Maintaining muscle speaks to our evolutionary development. Your body and brain were programmed to survive, and that's how your system still reacts. Stronger, leaner, faster—these qualities helped your prehistoric counterpart hunt down food, kill it, and eat it. There were no grocery stores, and because there were barriers to consumption, your forebear's body adapted to store energy in case food was unavailable for days or weeks. Today, the human body is still very adept at storing energy. The past hundred years mark the first time in human history that many of us haven't been living in a state of famine, which is all the more reason to maintain muscle mass. Muscle tissue helps regulate energy storage and consumption, determining how much weight you lose and how quickly.

Muscle is where much of the critical metabolic function happens—the more lean muscle you have, the more calories your body burns every day. Age-related muscle loss, known as sarcopenia, is one of the single greatest contributors to the human body's decline in function. The loss of muscle roughly parallels the decline in testosterone that typically occurs after age 30. Since testosterone is crucial to muscle building, it's harder to build and maintain muscle when you lose testosterone. Also, as you age, your force-generating type II (fast-twitch) muscle fibers begin to convert in the direction of type I (slow-twitch) muscle fibers, which may make you weaker, according to Joseph Signorile, PhD, in his book *Bending the Aging Curve*. In the aging man who doesn't exercise properly, loss of these fast-twitch muscle fibers conspires with a steady loss of collagen in your tendons as well as loss of bone mineral density, resulting in a lack of power, strength, and flexibility in activities that once seemed natural. Now you can see why a man in his eighties may have difficulty rising up out of a chair or car. What's worse is when a man in his sixties feels that way, and that can happen.

Even if your testosterone levels are optimized, you still need to do the resistance work to recover strength and power. By simply incorporating the right resistance exercises into your routine—specifically power moves, like plyometric jumps, deadlifts, pushups, and lunges—you will continue to build those important fast-twitch muscle fibers, the same ones that help you get out of a chair or push you up when you bend down to tie your shoes. Here's another benefit of weight-bearing resistance training: It produces a tugging impact on your skeleton, which stimulates your bones to lay down more bone cells and, over time, makes your infrastructure stronger.

My recommendation: Don't exercise to lose weight. Rather, exercise to build and maintain muscle, and then weight loss will follow. To build an effective exercise program, you must combine these essential components:

Resistance training: body-weight calisthenics and weight lifting

Balance: single-leg and single-arm exercises that challenge your core and full-body stability

Flexibility: static and dynamic stretches

Cardiovascular training: playing sports; doing explosive exercises like plyometrics (exercise without weights or machines); sprinting, running, rope jumping, or cycling; swimming, rowing, and other water sports; doing high-repetition weight lifting using light weights

Later in this chapter, I'll show you how to incorporate these four components into your exercise plan.

For now, acknowledge that you have an inner athlete, a body that's capable of high performance. Make no mistake: Your body was designed to move, and move a lot. To be at your healthiest, to avoid the disorders of aging, to sleep better, to strengthen your immune system, and to feel happier, you need to move every day. My recommendations will help orient you; over time, you will see how to incorporate all the key components most efficiently.

GETTING STARTED

You need to establish a routine for exercise, a series of steps that will help you achieve the muscle mass, balance, flexibility, strength, and cardiovascular endurance essential to "keep it up" to 100 and beyond.

So, let's start with the step-one prelude to any workout session: the warmup.

There's a reason athletes warm up before competition. It improves bloodflow, increases heart rate, boosts mental acuity, and lends an overall sense of well-being along with heightened energy. To prepare for your workout, I recommend foam rolling and dynamic warmups. This will reduce injuries and prime the body for movement, ultimately improving the quality of your workout.

Foam rolling is exactly as it sounds: You roll your muscles over a thick, firm tube of closed-cell foam. The goal is to relax the fascia, a sheath of thin connective tissue that surrounds the muscles, thereby allowing the muscle to expand. The fascia deserves attention because it affects function, flexibility, and performance. Remember, as you work out, bloodflow into the muscles increases, causing the muscles to grow in size. Foam rolling makes it easier for the soft tissue to extend, the muscle-to-tendon connection to stretch, and nerve-to-muscle messaging to be more efficient. All this reduces potential injuries. The bonus? You will feel better, with less pain in various muscle groups if you focus on foam rolling where you typically feel tight—calves, hamstrings, IT band (down the side of your upper leg), lower back, pecs, and lats. Once I started, my body quickly grew addicted to using the foam roller because it felt so good, before and after.

Foam rollers are offered in various lengths at most sporting goods stores or on fitness equipment Web sites. Buy one. It's like having a masseuse on call 24/7 for a one-time cost of less than $40.

Flexibility is the key component of most of our physical activities, both in the short and long term. Therefore, after you complete a foam-rolling session, I recommend what's known as a "dynamic warmup"—that is, doing active stretches like soldier kicks, scorpions, spiderman pushups, pigeon stretches, high-knee marches, fast-feet drills, slide and stretch drills, double touch skips, and arm circles. These calisthenics mimic the activities or exercises that will be performed later. Check KeepItUpTheBook.com for the dynamic warmup videos if you want to be sure you know the correct moves.

Foam rolling and a dynamic warmup will prime your body for the next steps: resistance training and cardio exercises. The two exercise physiologists on my staff, Steven Villagomez and Tim Coyle, recommend that our patients who are getting started, perform two to four resistance training sessions per week. They also suggest engaging in cardiovascular activity three to five times per week, though it doesn't have to be formal exercise. Just taking a brisk walk counts as good exercise.

I rarely recommend that people train for more than 40 minutes. Instead, you'll warm up, get ready for the workout, and then knock it out within 40 minutes. Why the short, intense session? There's an ideal window of adaptation for change to occur, after which the return on your investment of time diminishes. The kinds of exercises you do should vary from workout to workout, based on your current level of performance.

How should you structure your workouts? The answer depends on your individual needs, goals, and activity or sport of interest. You may benefit from consulting an educated, experienced, certified personal trainer to customize your exercise regimen and guide you as you transition and improve. A trainer can help you create a realistic timeline that starts in a general manner and allows you to work toward specific goals at various checkpoints in time. Alternatively, you may find local gyms that offer support, as well as helpful material online, in *Men's Health* magazine, and in its branded books. Feel free to get more details at KeepItUpTheBook.com.

CLIMBING THE FITNESS LADDER

The first 6 to 8 weeks of any exercise program, or any changes in your fitness routine, are mainly about mind-body connection. It's neurological training. I caution against going overboard on resistance training early on because you will be incredibly sore. And if you're sore, you won't want to work out again. Starting slow gives ligaments and tendons time to recover. Moreover, jumping into something intense like power lifting or rock climbing or just about any competitive sport without first training your body may—no, *will*—lead to injury. You don't want to be laid low with an injury just when you're ramping up. If you have a '65 Ferrari in the garage that hasn't been driven in 20 years, you wouldn't just fire her up and say, "Let's see how fast we can go." You'd get her back into shape.

We typically recommend that our patients begin with two resistance training sessions per week. That's what Steven recommended for Ethan B., my patient who's a high school principal and was embarrassed by how his body looked. (Ethan's story is in Chapter 4.) If you haven't been doing much resistance training, like Ethan, that's how you should start, too. Be sure to train both upper-body and lower-body muscles. Couple your exercise routine with a change in your diet, and as you increase your protein intake, resistance training will help strengthen the muscles in your body. The goal is to improve all of the tubing, all of the plumbing, the heart, and the organs. Maintaining the health of smooth muscle and skeletal muscle is the starting point, and this transition takes months. It took Ethan 3 months to incorporate changes so that he had a solid foundation upon which to build. Once you have this foundation, you can tailor your workouts to fit your expanded goals and needs. In the beginning, though, it's as much about training your brain to work in sync with your body. It will stop complaining after a while, really!

An educated, experienced, and certified trainer can be a huge help in planning an individualized (and safe) workout program, as well as correcting your form initially. You can also go it alone, and if you do, here are a few basics to get you started depending on your baseline level of fitness.

BEGINNER—PHASE 1

Aim to get in three to five workouts per week, and remember, only two of them should focus on resistance training. Note that I'm not talking about days per week, it's *sessions* I'm counting. In reality, you only have to be at the gym 3 days a week. You can do cardiovascular training and weight training on the same day. Additionally, I highly recommend doing your cardiovascular training in the morning on an empty stomach. If you train before breakfast, you will be able to burn any remaining sugar and fat stores. Working out before the morning meal, you won't have to deal with the insulin spike that occurs after you eat and can make you a little sluggish. If you combine your resistance and cardiovascular training, you'll want to save your aerobic activity for last. Tax your most immediate energy systems first.

THE SCIENCE OF MUSCLE 101

Today—and every day—you have the same number of muscle fibers as you did when you were born. That never changes. So you never really add muscle.

Resistance training breaks down muscle fiber, and acts primarily to rebuild type II muscle fibers. When the muscle repairs itself, the fibers grow bigger—providing they are getting proper nutrition. This process is known as hypertrophy, especially when tied to a specific type of resistance training. Type II muscle fibers make up glycolytic muscles, used by lifters.

If all you do is long-distance cardio, however, understand that you're training your muscles to get smaller. Why? Well, picture the needs of the long-distance runner: efficient muscles that are able to endure long-term exertion (type I muscle fibers). The more endurance training you do, the smaller the muscles become. These muscles are oxidative, meaning they need more oxygen to be pumped into them to function properly. They have a smaller cross-sectional area (relative to type II) and they don't generate a lot of force. That's why you see skinny marathon runners and muscular, lean sprinters: two different muscle requirements, two different kinds of training. If you want your muscles to grow, endurance training alone is the wrong way to go.

A NOTE OF CAUTION TO THE SEDENTARY OR UNCONDITIONED: Depending on your state of health and your risk factors, such as high blood pressure, your doctor will usually want to do a physical examination and an EKG before you launch into a new fitness regimen. For some men, a stress test may be recommended. In most cases, if your situation is not dire your doctor will tell you to go forward as you wish. Don't embark on any new exercise routine until your doctor gives you the green light.

If you are hypertensive (that is, have high blood pressure), do not do resistance training until your cardiologist says your blood pressure is low enough to tolerate it. You may need to focus first on improving cardiovascular function. With proper guidance, however, a mild form of resistance training may provide some peripheral adaptations (changes) to help relieve pressure on your heart. This type of resistance training involves light weights and repetitions in the 15 to 25 range so that your movements mimic cardiovascular activity. Light cardio that uses your whole body (such as swimming, using a rowing machine, or even walking) is a good option.

Many of us view walking only as a mode of transportation; however, it is a good place to start. After a few weeks of walking, you will want to do more, because you will feel better as you go forward. As your body gets stronger, you'll notice that your recovery is quicker. Pay attention, then ramp up your activity as advised. If you start as a beginner, it will take about 10 to 12 weeks to adapt to your new routine.

INTERMEDIATE—PHASE 2

Many people fall into this middle group. As a general rule, if you're exercising around three to five times a week (remember, I'm counting sessions, not days), then you may be at this intermediate level. The goal here is to get serious and take it up a notch. To reach a new level of fitness, you need to raise the level of intensity and at the same time decrease the volume (the time spent training). You should increase your resistance training to three sessions weekly. Also schedule three cardiovascular sessions, with one longer classic aerobic session (like a long run) and two interval-training sessions.

Interval is a fancy word for sprint training. You work at a rate that's above your anaerobic threshold, where you're burning mostly carbohydrates, which have been stored as glycogen in your muscles. That means you're burning the gas in your gas tank—a good thing, because you want your body to become better at burning all of its various types of fuel. As your body burns this fuel and goes through this process termed anaerobic glycolysis, you will produce lactic acid in your muscles. That's what gives your muscles that burning sensation during exercise. It's a powerful molecular signal telling the body, *Look, we've been stressed, we need to adapt*, so testosterone and growth hormone are released from that type of training. Again, that's a good thing. Testosterone and growth hormone allow your body to repair and strengthen muscle fiber.

Interval training is simple: It's about the work-to-rest ratio. Let's say you sprint for 30 seconds, then go at a light pace for 1 minute, then sprint for 30, and so on. So, in this case work to recovery ratio is 1 to 2. At this intermediate level, you might be exhausted after 10 minutes (maybe even less). That's okay. You want a stark difference between the two paces. The more frequently you interval train per week (up to three or four sessions), the more fit you will become. The fitter you are, the harder you can work and the longer you will have to rest between spurts of activity. *One important note:* Have a solid foundation in cardiovascular training before you attempt interval training. You can adjust the work-to-rest ratio depending on your training status. For example, try 5 to 10 seconds of sprinting (like a 40-yard dash or 100-meter sprint) and 90 seconds to 3 minutes of rest. Various types of exercise lend themselves to interval training, including rowing, cycling, and swimming. Also, most intense competitive sports—like basketball, soccer, rugby, even ultimate Frisbee—mimic interval training.

I recommend interval training for endurance athletes, too. You'll get similar results while preventing over-training. It is also good for improving speed. Why? Simply put, your muscles adapt to the speed at which you train them. If you're going for, say, a 45-minute jog, cortisol runs high, blocking pathways for growth hormone or testosterone. What does that mean in the bigger scheme of things? Imagine you're going to remodel your house. Longer cardiovascular training, let's say a 2-hour run, is like having 10 guys come to do the demo work (cortisol) and no one shows up to do the reconstruction (testosterone and growth hormone). You're breaking yourself down, consistently. With interval training, you'll have a hormonal response where your body produces growth hormone and testosterone—which is like having 5 guys demolishing the house and 10 guys rebuilding it better than it was previously. You're maintaining that level of endurance, but you're getting stronger, too. The point once again being, I want you to ramp up the intensity of your workouts, not necessarily the volume. Go short and intense, not long and slow, for a more productive workout.

When Wayne Hickory got a personal trainer to help keep him on track with his exercise routine, I recommended they focus on interval training. Wayne travels a lot, and interval training is an attractive choice when you're tight on time.

> Interval training is where they claim you have the greatest benefit per unit of time. We only have just so much time to exercise, and if you're on something steady like the treadmill, you're not going to get as much conditioning as you do with intervals. They've shown that interval training also burns the most calories. What we do is just a minute or two of one exercise, and then we step back and do something else. I'm constantly engaged and being challenged.
>
> **—WAYNE HICKORY,** orthodontist

Your performance will rise with the amount of interval training you do. Most important, your resting heart rate will decrease. Your heart will get stronger and be more likely to respond to exercise in a positive way, increasing the amount of available oxygen for your coronary arteries at a faster rate. This is especially important if you're facing an acute stress, which might otherwise result in a heart attack. As your heart becomes a more efficient pump, your heart muscle cells (called myocytes) will get the oxygen they need to survive. Remember: You don't want to jump right into intense interval training if you've been sedentary or haven't been doing any cardiovascular exercise. Your body may not be able to withstand such a strain on its vasculature. Start slowly with cardio. When you are ready to try interval training, expect to take about 10 to 12 weeks to adapt to your new routine. Once you are comfortable, make it more challenging.

EXPERT—PHASE 3

If you're a well-trained competitive athlete, you know what your body needs. I do have several suggestions of my own:

IF YOU ENJOY A SPORT, KEEP DOING IT. A lot of men play competitive sports and continue throughout their lives, as John Bellizzi does with soccer. Others may play when they're young, drift away, and then suddenly decide to return to that sport when they hit 40 or beyond. They often get hurt jumping in suddenly. If you decide to reengage, do it slowly. Practice. Train your body. Remember: It's a lot easier to stay in shape than it is to get back in shape.

CROSS-TRAIN. If you devote a lot of time to one sport or activity, take a break once a week to do something else. The variety will help you in the long term. This is especially important as you age. Take running, for example. Running is brutal on aging joints, so switching up to a low-impact activity like swimming or cycling is a great way to keep your muscles challenged while giving your body a break from pounding the pavement.

IMPROVE YOUR NUTRITION. You may need further increases in protein and in calories overall. Many high-level athletes consume 1.4 to 1.6 grams of protein per kilogram of body weight per day and, depending on the sport, sometimes more. Many of my male patients who are expert athletes do not consume enough to maintain or increase muscle. At this level, you're likely quite knowledgeable about your energy levels and requirements. Nevertheless, if you notice changes in your body despite the care and attention you're giving it, revisit your personal metrics. There may be a clue in your family history that you previously overlooked, or a critical component of your lifestyle that you've neglected lately (sleep, for example).

ADJUST CARDIOVASCULAR TRAINING. Increase the intensity of cardiovascular training and further reduce the volume. I highly recommend doing Tabata-style cardio after every resistance-training session, plus one long aerobic session per week. Tabata follows an interval-training format, using a 2 to 1 work-to-rest ratio. Most commonly, this entails 20 seconds of active work followed by 10 seconds recovery, repeated in succession 8 to 20 times.

Remember Marvin Lagstein from Chapter 3? He was in his late sixties and running too much. In terms of muscle, the majority of what he was using was type I. This marathoner's makeup, however, was doing tremendous damage to his bones. Despite getting test results that confirmed that he was osteoporotic with fragile bones, with evidence of stress fractures (thin visible breaks), Marvin resisted switching up his routine. It took him a year to begin following my recommendations. Then he combined resistance training to strengthen his bones with a type of aerobic exercise that wouldn't break down his body. Marvin started pace training, and has continued to do well over the past 4 years.

Juxtapose Marvin's story with that of Livingston Miller's (Chapter 1), and you'll see both ends of the fitness spectrum. Before he came to my office, Livingston was literally the poster child for fitness. As the model for the New York City gym he worked at, Livingston was featured on advertisements posted on bus stop kiosks and in Grand Central Terminal. A Jamaican man in his fifties, Livingston looked at least a decade younger, thanks to his physique: nearly 210 pounds of solid muscle. He had served in the US Army as a unit drill instructor. He had been a fitness coach for 6 years and was now working as a personal trainer. By all accounts, he appeared to be in great shape.

Yet between teaching classes and training clients in addition to working out on his own, he was too focused on resistance training. Livingston was consistently working his type II muscles.

When my resident exercise physiologist, Steven, put Livingston through our VO_2 assessment test (see Chapter 10), there was a disconnect between his athletic lifestyle and his results. After he cycled for a few minutes, I could see that his lung capacity was not optimal and his heart rate was too low, not able to keep up with the demands of the physical activity he was performing. I referred him to a cardiologist, who found that Livingston had what's known as left anterior wall hypokinesis. The test result suggested that Livingston may have already experienced a silent heart attack. Having this cardiac defect is like using a four-cylinder engine to power a Mack truck. It's greatly limiting, and all of Livingston's excess muscle mass was putting more strain on his heart as well.

When I made my recommendations to Livingston, I didn't ask him to abandon his resistance training. In fact, I aim to never use the words *eliminate* or *abandon*. Instead, I suggested that he increase his aerobic training and rely less on the hypertrophy model, which is classic in body-building routines. Now Livingston is down 20 pounds of muscle and body fat, and his heart doesn't have to work as hard to supply blood to body tissue that ultimately wasn't necessary for him anyway.

Looking at Marvin and Livingston, it just goes to show that even people who look very healthy may not be. You may have to change your fitness routine not only to get better results at the gym but also to safe-guard your health.

GETTING REAL

DON'T TRY TO CHANGE MORE THAN THREE HABITS IN A MONTH. You shouldn't expect to change everything at once. I think this is important to empha-size, and it reinforces our process approach to health. It's always going to be journey. Even when you get healthier, it remains a balancing act, and you will continue to make adjustments in order to improve further.

Success depends on how willing you are to change your habits. The more sedentary folks are usually the most challenged, though not always. If you are an athlete who is set in your routine, it may be hard to switch it up. It is not impossible, however. You can adjust slowly, over time, just like Marvin. I like to "add one, subtract one" if you tend to be more resis-tant to change. You might opt to select an activity or exercise in that case.

The Lost Athlete

Dave M., a former college football star, was an impatient kind of patient. From the moment he started the program, Dave wanted to measure his progress in numbers and craved constant feedback. He was the alpha bull, used to having a coach yelling in his face. His total cholesterol, LDL, and triglycerides were all very high, and even though he was battling a knee injury, he was still dreaming of competing athletically.

In May 2012, however, Dave was growing a little discouraged. He didn't have a sport to call his own, and he didn't think his blood work numbers were where they should be given the changes he was making to his diet and exercise routine. He demanded results, and began preoccupying himself with his weight. He was a solid 200-something pound man.

Even with his not-so-great lipid panel, my exercise physiologist, Steven, showed Dave that he had improved at an average or above-average pace precisely because he has that athletic drive. Still, his body composition (muscle and fat) showed that he was 21.5 percent fat, too high. Dave had been taught as a football player to maintain as much mass as possible. Now he wanted to drop pounds. To see results, he would need to lose both muscle and fat.

We talked about it and decided that the best way for him to lose mass (fat and muscle) was to use a lot of both of them. My exercise physiologist Tim suggested Dave find a new sport to practice regularly, to which Dave responded that he was going to begin training for an Olympic-distance triathlon, consisting of a swim of almost a mile, then a bike ride of 25 miles, and finishing with a run of 6.2 miles. The training for such an endurance race requires proper planning and constant tweaking. Dave would also have to be careful not to overtrain. Muscular strength is not so easily lost; however, endurance capability requires regularity with regard to training and can disappear much more rapidly.

Given that Dave played strong safety on his college football team, he was used to barreling straight into tough challenges. He assumed he would be ready to go in 4 months, and we admired his commitment. We did suggest that he use a coach. Dave did the research on his own and found one nearby; now we get his training results through a GPS tracking system. Soon after the first meeting, Dave's coach was the one who suggested he scale back his expectations. Still, Dave competed in a half-marathon in January 2013. That April, he completed the Alcatraz swim, in which competitors swim from Alcatraz Island to the California mainland. Soon he hopes to do that Olympic-distance triathlon.

As you progress in your training, you can begin ramping up a bit faster. Some men can establish a habit in 2 weeks, and for others it takes longer. The first step is awareness coupled with the desire to change.

WEAR A HEART MONITOR. Keep track of your heart rate as it rises. As you become better conditioned, you'll be able to walk faster and cover more distance in the same amount of time at the same heart rate. This is good: It means your heart is getting stronger.

KEEP THE TESTOSTERONE FLOWING. No matter what your sport or skill level, practice interval and resistance training for all the reasons I've mentioned. Both types of exercise help your body produce more of its own testosterone and growth hormone, necessary for muscles to grow. This is crucial as you age because your muscles will naturally atrophy in the absence of activity. Regular, disciplined training is the only way you'll ever be able to regain and maintain an athletic (and bedroom) performance that will keep you vital and make you smile.

Now lace up and get out there!

CHAPTER 8

VITAMINS AND DIETARY SUPPLEMENTS

Even if you eat like a nutritionist, consider investing in supplemental insurance

Dr. Comite gave me supplements and told me why she wanted me to take them. She didn't just say, "Take fish oil." She told me how each supplement would impact the values on my blood tests. So, there was always a "what?" and a "why?" and a "how are we going to solve it?" The knowledge I've gotten from working with her enables me to stay committed. I understand what happens when I don't. For example, I fell off the wagon with supplements. I had a busy travel schedule and ran out of them several weeks before my next scheduled blood tests. My first instinct was to go back on them quickly and cheat so I wouldn't get in trouble. But I didn't cheat, and you could see the difference in the blood work. To me, that was direct proof to dispel the myth around whether or not vitamins work.

—**ERAN KABAKOV,** age 39, physical therapist and digital entrepreneur

B alance is everything in maintaining a good quality of life, and it's not simple. The preceding chapters have targeted key areas that deserve attention. Improvements in your sleep quality, stress level, sex life, diet plan, and exercise routine are critical. Additionally, there's something else you can do to support your health: Consider taking certain dietary supplements to ensure that you are compensating for critical nutrients that you may not be getting enough from the foods you eat.

Supplements should not be taken randomly. You must be selective about which dietary additions you need and be consistent in taking them. Supplements typically don't work like caffeine, providing you with an instantaneous perceptible boost. Rather, over a period of regular use, you will feel the benefit. It could be when you first wake up, during a workout, at the end of your workday, or at night, helping you to sleep. Supplements provide you with the vitamins and minerals that are the key drivers of many of your body's processes.

Why is supplementation important? Well, you no longer live in a simple environment and culture where you know the sources of your food. Unless you're shopping at a local farmers' market (and even then, it's tough to ascertain how the food was grown and handled), you'll be getting apples ripened in cold storage and tomatoes picked when they were green—in other words, food that hasn't been allowed to ripen to its nutritional potential. You're not going to get the food that will keep you at your healthiest in every respect. Most of you aren't growing your own produce in your own backyards. Even if you did, the soil doesn't have the same nutrients it had 100 or even 50 years ago. This may impact the quality of the food grown in it. Modern society has created a nutrition gap that supplements may help fill. Don't think that supplements should replace meals; rather, they should provide additional elements that help fill in the holes.

Caution: Even though most are available over the counter without a prescription, supplements should ideally be taken under the guidance of a physician. Many supplements and medications taken together may create negative interactions. Also, it is possible to go overboard in terms of supplementation. I make my recommendations for patients based on their personal health metrics, my aim being to lower systemic inflammation. I can track this by looking at measures like homocysteine and c-CRP, and how they respond over time while a patient is taking a customized blend of supplements.

WHAT'S IN YOUR SUPPLEMENTS?

This chapter won't provide a list of supplements that "everybody" should take. No two people live the same way; no two people have identical nutritional needs. What works for your friends may not work for you. Instead, this chapter offers groupings of supplements to consider in consultation with your doctor. They are organized based on their effect on the body.

When managed properly, supplements can be a great addition to a healthy lifestyle. Some of my patients like to test approaches and interventions the way they would if participating in a research study, meaning that they change one thing at a time and see how that works for them. That's often how I like to operate, particularly if allergies are a concern. Other patients I see, however, are so sick of feeling low that they add several supplements at once, hoping to make significant gains quickly. You will have to proceed at the pace that feels right for you. Remember, our focus here is on continued progress and prevention, not quick fixes or magic pills.

I base my recommendations on my clinical experience in synchrony with an individual's makeup. These recommendations are further grounded in published research, and I suggest brands I know have been tested for quality. Manufacturing processes vary, and it's especially important with regard to supplements that you get the ingredients you want. Understand that supplements are not regulated by the Food and Drug Administration. As such, you need to be extra cautious. Beware of labels that read like infomercials, heavy on the hyperbole.

Because there is no regulatory body enforcing the source, activity, absorption, manufacture, and labeling of supplements, you could be buying something that's inactive or even toxic. This shouldn't scare you off. It should simply make you more vigilant and inquisitive when shopping at stores and especially online. Keep in mind that sales staff in various health food outlets may not be formally trained on the specifics of supplements; they may be incentivized to sell certain products, not necessarily those that are best for you. As a rule, search for supplements that contain a certificate of analysis whenever possible. This means that the company has tested that specific batch of supplements to ensure the only ingredients it contains are the ones you see listed on the container and in the stated amounts. Right now, a certificate of analysis is the closest you'll get to being certain of what you are putting in your body.

Truth be told, it's overwhelming to walk down an aisle in your local pharmacy and figure out supplements. My medical training did not teach me about supplements, so for a long time I was reluctant to even recommend them to my patients. In the 1980s and early '90s, I kept the brochures describing greens and fruit powder supplements in my office closet, sharing selectively with patients who asked me questions. My opinion soon began to shift after one of my medical school classmates (Dr. Candace Corson, always ahead of the curve with regard to natural health approaches) gave me a couple of posters from the American Cancer Society and American Heart Association that explained the value of produce and of eating all the colors of the rainbow. It was then that I began to mention to patients the benefit of utilizing supplements when it is not possible to get enough healthy foods. Still, it gave me pause. I didn't actually change my mind until I was faced with a problem in my immediate family. One of my sons was not eating a healthy diet, and I was concerned about his growth and development, especially since it was tough to get him to exercise. After I began to review the available research, my focus shifted to determining the value of supplements in the same way as I evaluate FDA-approved medications. Over the years, I have worked to ensure that my recommendations take into account all critical factors, such as effectiveness and sourcing, as well as the individual nature of each patient.

I look for options to facilitate supplement use by combining a variety of nutrients, beyond multivitamins, that are active and bioavailable. It is important to cherry-pick the various nutrients you need; nevertheless, I have found that certain supplements benefit most men across the board. My clinical experience has allowed me to create customized blends.

Personally, I don't like to take many pills. It can be annoying and time consuming, adding more burdens to an already busy life. In recent years, I have worked with a lab in Germany to formulate highly bioavailable supplement blends called BioG MicroTabs that support systemic health instead of managing just one symptom. With every shipment of BioG MicroTabs I receive a certificate of analysis for *each individual ingredient from each blend.* My patients and I know exactly what is in each jar. The preparations I recommend to most patients are called Prime Alpha, Prime Alpha Plus, Prime Power, Prime Strength, and Prime Immunity, sold under my proprietary brand FloQi. Prime Alpha and Prime Alpha Plus promote vascular flow. Prime Power has, to me, redefined the multivitamin. I formulated it to combine with Prime Strength, which is geared toward promoting bone, muscle, and joint health, combining several additional antioxidants, anti-inflammatories, vitamins, and nutrients. Prime Immunity is loaded with antioxidants. These custom blends are ideal for men who have trouble taking pills, no matter the size. You swallow a capful or more of these tiny tabs, much like the size of those colorful flash-frozen ice-cream bits. This delivery method allows for faster release and less irritation of the stomach and intestines. You don't want to chew MicroTabs. It's best to take the tabs with water or flavored seltzer, just like regular pills. One of our patients enjoys taking his MicroTabs with a chaser of a virgin Bloody Mary! Others take them mixed in a tablespoon of yogurt. FloQi supplements are available in capsules that are filled with MicroTabs and are relatively small in size. Some people find capsules easier, especially when on the road. Taking several at once is not difficult for me.

HOW TO SAMPLE AND USE SUPPLEMENTS

Treat supplements as seriously as you would a prescription medication. To the best of your abilities, collect all the unique medical information that makes you, you. Review it with your personal doctor to determine what you need. Discuss what dosage and frequency will help you most. Then track your results over time.

Your lab results should reflect your adherence to supplementation program. If you are taking a supplement and not seeing corresponding improvements in your lab measures, it may indicate a lifestyle problem, a persistent bad habit. Other possibilities are that you may not be absorbing the supplement properly, the dose may be inadequate, or you may need another element to complement the first supplement. For example, if you are taking vitamin D_2, yet your lab data still shows low vitamin D levels, then I recommend eating foods or taking supplements containing prebiotics which help the gut-friendly bacteria flourish, and probiotics, which often improve digestive absorption.

What follows is a mini-glossary of the supplements I most frequently recommend for reducing oxidative stress and improving immunity, optimizing metabolism and hormone function, and strengthening physical performance.

SUPPLEMENTS FOR REDUCING OXIDATIVE STRESS AND BOOSTING IMMUNITY

Oxidative stress is the leading cause of cardiovascular disease. You've heard of "free radicals." These are reactive oxygen particles triggered by inflammation and the daily natural processes of living. These free radicals damage our DNA; specifically, they are what cause our telomeres to shorten. Think of telomeres as tips of shoelaces—they're the ends of your DNA strands, which fray and pull apart with age as well as basic wear and tear, impacted by your lifestyle choices. Shortening of the telomeres leads to poor cell lines that are susceptible to disease. More on telomeres in Chapter 12.

L-ARGININE. You can combat oxidative stress and chronic inflammation by utilizing antioxidant vitamins and anti-inflammatories, such as L-arginine. L-arginine is a nonessential amino acid, meaning it can be made by your body from L-citrulline. However, the amounts of arginine and citrulline your body makes are not enough to be considered therapeutic, so I pair the two in a supplement. L-arginine stimulates nitric oxide production in the endothelium, the thin inner lining of the arteries. Nitric oxide is released into the blood vessels and promotes vasodilation—the opening or widening of the blood vessels. It keeps plaque from adhering to artery walls. What's more, nitric oxide helps you to get an erection.

VITAMIN B$_6$, FOLATE (VITAMIN B$_9$), AND VITAMIN B$_{12}$. The B-complex vitamins are vital in controlling chronic inflammation. The complex can help lower homocysteine, a marker of inflammation. If it's too high, homocysteine may indicate damage in your blood vessels, putting you at increased risk for heart disease. Eating enough fruits and vegetables may give you some benefit. However, to keep homocysteine down, you will likely need to supplement with B vitamins.

VITAMINS C AND E. These potent antioxidants help remove free radicals from your cells and improve immune system function. This is why products such as Airborne and Emergen-C are so popular. Loading up on vitamin C intake before hopping on an airplane might help you avoid picking up a bug. Vitamins C (as well as E) are also effective in exercise recovery, since your body's reaction to exercise is essentially an immune response that elicits short-term inflammation, triggering later beneficial adaptations like increased stamina and lean muscle mass.

Even though ongoing supplementation is often helpful, long-term overuse of vitamin C can lead to resistance that decreases the ability of antioxidants to remove free radicals from your cells. It is best to get your vitamin C through food, then consider supplementation, especially if you are very active. Or, if you or people around you are getting sick, that's a good time to turn to supplements to boost immune support. My Prime Immunity blend of BioG MicroTabs is formulated for patients to take for 7 days when they are not well, or when they undergo a significant lifestyle change like starting an exercise program.

Vitamin E is a common ingredient in lotions and skin care products. Found also in food, including certain vegetables and fruit, as well as almonds, it acts as an antioxidant inside your body. There are several useful, tocopherol versions of vitamin E; alphatocopherol is the most bioavailable form. Vitamin E is also indicated to help concentration, improve performance and energy levels, hasten the healing of wounds, normalize blood pressure, and ameliorate the damage caused by atherosclerosis, oxidative stress, and inflammation. Vitamin E is fat-soluble, meaning it is best absorbed in the presence of fatty acids.

OMEGA-3 FATTY ACIDS. When using vitamin E, be sure to supplement with the omega-3 fatty acids DHA (docosahexaenoic acid) and EPA (eicosapentaenoic acid), the main difference between the two being molecular structure. As you may remember, these were covered in Chapter 7. Later in this chapter, I'll discuss omegas from the perspective of performance. Supporting a number of physiological processes, they definitely go hand in hand with offsetting oxidative stress as well as metabolic and hormonal optimization.

VITAMIN D. As you know from Chapter 4, you need plenty of this hormone as you age for bone maintenance and metabolic function. There is mounting evidence that vitamin D deficiency in elderly people is a silent epidemic that results in bone loss and fractures, and that subadequate levels contribute to the risk of immunologic disorders, cancer, and cardiovascular disease.

DARK CHOCOLATE. For some of you, labeling chocolate as a supplement may be a stretch; however, it happens to be my favorite choice on a daily basis. I have been following the research on dark chocolate for years. The good news is that it is an extremely potent antioxidant. Raw, unprocessed cocoa has the highest oxygen radical absorbance capacity (ORAC). ORAC is a method of measuring antioxidant capacities in biological samples. Dark chocolate—and I mean the deep, dark, bitter stuff—is full of antioxidants and can lower your blood pressure.

In fact, dark chocolate with a cocoa content of 75 percent and higher has more antioxidants than blueberries.

Here are the benefits of eating 1 ounce of dark chocolate a day:

- You might get a little thinner: A study published in *Archives of Internal Medicine* indicates that frequent consumption of chocolate (at least two times a week) was associated with a lower body mass index.

- You could be protected from heart disease: Several studies connect the high flavonoid content of dark chocolate with protection from atherosclerosis (hardening of the arteries), ischemic heart disease, heart failure, and carotid artery plaque.

- You might slow the aging process: Dark chocolate is loaded with antioxidants, which protect from heart disease, some cancers, and the ravages of aging at a cellular level.

You might be disappointed to learn that milk or white chocolate does not yield the same benefits as the dark stuff. Generally, any chocolate bar out of the vending machine is a no go.

GREENS AND FRUIT POWDERS. Commercially prepared mixtures of extracts from fruits, including berries and vegetables, are available in a powder that you mix in beverages. But Dr. Corson suggested the capsules and soft chewables known as Juice Plus+. These can provide nutrients that are essential to the healthy function of your body and mind. As you increase your activity in the gym, your body demands quality fuel. Working out will increase oxidative stress, and homocysteine may rise as you become more active. Your body is revving up, demanding more nutrients, and thus you need more antioxidants to counter the stress. I typically ask my patients to eat a variety of vegetables and fruits in salads and as snacks throughout the day. To make sure my patients get the nutrients they might be missing and because many expressed an interest in cutting down on their pill load, I've added greens and fruit powders to the Prime Power MicroTab preparation. Now, most of my patients supplement with Prime Power in addition to maintaining a healthy diet rich in low-glycemic raw vegetables and fruits.

GREEN TEA EXTRACT. Green tea extract is one of the best sources of anti-oxidants, which are important because they counter free radicals, the primary contributors to aging. Green tea extract can help rev up your metabolism, boost cardiovascular health and energy levels, and even improve skin quality. Just keep an eye on the label. Avoid products that include sugar, artificial sweeteners, preservatives, alcohol, gluten or calories.

MELATONIN. You may remember from Chapter 5 that the hormone melatonin decreases with aging, even though this hormone is useful to regulate sleep. Melatonin will help you get to sleep and stay asleep. It is a powerful antioxidant, even in tiny doses. Some folks find that it helps mitigate the effects of jet lag and so they take it when traveling. Doses can be quite variable, starting at less than 1 milligram and increasing to more than 20 milligrams. Men have reported grogginess with even tiny amounts, so I recommend starting small and increasing slowly.

RESVERATROL. Resveratrol in capsule form is not a supplement that I commonly recommend, since I find most patients are likely consuming it regularly. Many people believe red wine is good for you because of its resveratrol content. Found in the skin of red grapes, resveratrol is known for its antioxidant properties, shielding the body from damage. You would never be able to drink enough wine, though, to reap the benefits of the widely accepted recommendation of 400 milligrams daily of resveratrol. (You would die of alcohol poisoning well before your 40th bottle.) It's possible that a bit of resveratrol, consistently consumed over time may benefit you, though research has indicated that wine drinkers are in better health in general when compared to beer and liquor drinkers. This is due to socioeconomic reasons, not necessarily because of wine's health benefits.

SELENIUM. Men need this trace mineral to produce sperm, and selenium is also linked to prostate cancer prevention. It may ward off lung cancer and could help alleviate symptoms of diabetes. Two great natural selenium sources are Brazil nuts and meat. At higher doses, however, selenium supplementation may reduce the effectiveness of statins and decrease vitamin C absorption.

SUPPLEMENTS FOR METABOLIC AND HORMONAL OPTIMIZATION

Metabolic and hormonal optimization is at the heart of all of your body's processes, so you'll notice that some supplements overlap between this section and others. Each of you is a complex system with many branches that connect to your core. So even though you may be taking a B vitamin in the hopes of improving your homocysteine, which is a very targeted outcome, that same supplement may also have a more general effect by improving your cognition and boosting energy levels. Remember, metabolism is the mechanism by which your body turns chemical energy into mechanical energy, and hormones drive this process. Supplements may assist both metabolic and hormonal aspects to function optimally.

CONJUGATED LINOLEIC ACID. CLA has been shown to have a positive impact on coronary artery disease risk factors, and there are studies that suggest CLA is useful for weight loss, particularly in those individuals who are exercising regularly.

VITAMIN D. In addition to its immunity-boosting properties, vitamin D is hugely important in metabolic and hormonal optimization because it is involved in insulin sensitivity. Supplementing with D may increase the body's sensitivity to insulin, helping men with type 2 diabetes and insulin resistance. Your body also requires vitamin D for your bones to properly absorb calcium and thus prevent osteopenia and osteoporosis. Vitamin D also helps regulate how much calcium and phosphorus—two elements essential to muscle contraction—circulate in your bloodstream. Calcium and phosphate are usually plentiful on their own when you eat well. Still, vitamin D supplementation may positively affect their concentration in your blood. As I mentioned in Chapter 4, there are two types of vitamin D supplements. Look for vitamin D_3, which is available over the counter, or get a prescription from your doctor for D_2. Some men are better able to absorb D_2.

PROBIOTICS. The healthy bacteria in probiotics can aid digestion and absorption of nutrients—especially the nutrient supplements recommended here. A healthy GI tract is loaded with good bacteria that can be depleted by antibiotics (*pro*biotic, *anti*biotic; see the connection?) as well as by environmental and food toxins. You need these bacteria to line the surface of your intestine so that when food passes through, they help your intestines absorb the nutrients. The typical person has about 5 pounds of bacteria in his or her stomach. Prebiotics (indirectly) and probiotics can repopulate your gut with bacteria. Prebiotics have recently (in 1995) been identified as non-digestible food ingredients that are thought to have a beneficial effect on the digestive system as they stimulate the growth and activity of bacteria. Bacteria that live in symbiosis with your digestive system ensure that nutrients are digested and absorbed. Also, as you age, the enzymes in your stomach that aid in the nutrient-absorption process decrease. Digestive enzymes can often help if symptoms of malabsorption or discomfort during digestion are present.

SUPPLEMENTS FOR PERFORMANCE: MENTAL, PHYSICAL, SEXUAL

I eat well, but supplements also play an important role. I have been on arginine for more than 4 years and can say it definitely improves my workouts and overall quality of life. I usually wake up at 5:30 a.m., take my supplements along with a protein shake at 5:45 a.m., and then work out at 6:30 a.m.; I have another protein shake after the workout, which covers me until either a light breakfast or early lunch. In a perfect world, I would wake up and have a big meal, then work out, but I do not know anyone who has the time for that.

—**MIKE SENFT,** age 54, investment banker

When it comes to performance, certain supplements can really give you an edge, whether it is mental, physical, sexual, or a combination of the aforementioned. I've touched on some of these supplements earlier, yet here you'll see them in a new light.

L-ARGININE. As you read in the section on oxidative stress and immunity, L-arginine can help relax blood vessels. Vasodilation occurs throughout your entire arterial tree and can positively impact erectile function. It can improve libido in men, too. L-arginine is also beneficial before exercise. Taken 1 hour prior to your workout, no matter whether you're doing aerobic or resistance training, arginine increases bloodflow by carrying a greater amount of oxygen and nutrients to the working muscles. Combine this with an adequate amount of cardiovascular activity and you may increase your capillary density. As the smallest blood vessels in your body, the capillaries are the points of exchange between the arteries and muscles. L-citrulline is paired with arginine to replenish arginine quickly within the endothelial cells that line your blood vessels. Meanwhile, L-citrulline helps to rid the body of lactic acid, a by-product of strenuous, anaerobic muscle activity.

Many men report an increase in thirst with arginine use because their vascular system expands. This is a good sign that you are actually absorbing the arginine. More often than not, I ramp my patients up gradually because some people are more sensitive to this supplement's effects than others. A good starting point is 1 or 2 grams of arginine with 0.5 or 1 gram of citrulline. Ingesting the combination along with caffeine or coffee is a great way to boost your workouts.

Another combination of L-arginine and L-citrulline with L-ornithine is recommended prior to sleep. Ornithine is involved in resynthesizing arginine so that you continue receiving the positive effects during the night. This may augment the body's ability to lose weight, improve muscular performance, and increase nitric oxide production. Remember, nitric oxide is produced by your body to help in vasodilation (opening blood vessels wider), which aids bloodflow to your brain, heart, muscles, and penis. A number of supplement companies market nitric oxide supplements for these functions. L-arginine, however, *naturally* promotes your body's own physiological processes for vasodilation. The direct supplementation of nitric oxide can shut down your body's own production. A similar thing happens when you undergo testosterone treatment, and the brain stops sending the signals to your testes to manufacture testosterone because there appears to be adequate amounts circulating through your body.

B-COMPLEX VITAMINS. If food is your fuel, then B-complex vitamins are high-grade oil helping your engine run better. B vitamins assist with almost every process in your body, including healthy digestion; a strong nervous system; good hair, skin, and nails; and energy production. That's because B vitamins help convert carbohydrates into glucose. This sugar is then converted by your body into energy (or, if you're not active enough or have poor glucose metabolism, fat). If you overindulge in alcohol, you need B replenishment because alcohol depletes it. Niacin is a popular choice of oral B-supplementation among many because it's been reported to increase HDL, or good cholesterol. I have also found that a supplement called HDL-Rx has boosted HDL in some of our patients.

Note: Some vitamins, like B_{12}, are not easily absorbed from the stomach and may need to be taken by injection periodically or via nasal spray. Your doctor can advise you on options. Injection or spray forms of B vitamins like niacin need to be prescribed. Don't fear the needle: We employ a very small and thin needle on an insulin syringe, which my patients find painless and easy for use at home.

One of the things that came up in my family medical history was high cholesterol and heart disease, and my blood work showed that my cholesterol wasn't great. My HDL was low. After I started taking niacin, on the second blood draw 3 months later, my HDL was better. It slowly has been getting better and better because of the combination of the niacin and everything else I'm doing. Just because I don't feel this breakdown happening and the diseases that are creeping up quietly doesn't mean it's not a real threat. To be able to do that blood draw and see the effect of the niacin on my HDL and the effect of the B vitamins on my energy level really put it in perspective.

—ERAN KABAKOV

CAFFEINE. Everyone knows that caffeine boosts energy. But studies show that it's particularly good for improving performance with long-duration exercise; two to six cups of coffee taken about 60 minutes before intense exercise seems to work best. The healthiest way to take caffeine, I've found, is through drinking coffee and tea because those drinks also contain powerful polyphenols. Longitudinal studies (research conducted over time) have shown that people who drink up to six cups of coffee daily actually have a decreased risk of diabetes and a better chance of living longer.

I tell patients to drink coffee or tea before exercise, especially if they usually drink it anyway. In physically fit individuals with larger, more dense mitochondria, caffeine aids in fat breakdown, increasing the delivery of glucose to be used as energy. This especially helps those who want to lose weight. Caffeine increases mental alertness and acuity and improves mood. While caffeine or coffee is viewed as a diuretic, hydration depletion is less profound than widely believed. Besides, you should be drinking enough water to not have to worry about this effect.

COENZYME Q10 (CoQ10). Produced by the body, CoQ10 is necessary for the basic function of cells. It is essential for mitochondrial function—the energy producers of each cell in your body. Organs with the highest energy needs—the heart, liver, and kidneys, for example—have the highest concentration of CoQ10. Statins, one of the most commonly prescribed drugs, lower these levels. If you are on a statin, you'll likely need to supplement with CoQ10. In my experience, the muscle cramps many people experience on statins are less likely with the complementary use of CoQ10.

CREATINE. Supplementing with creatine is not recommended, except perhaps, for elite high-level athletes. Your body likely makes enough of this chemical on its own to produce the right amount of muscle mass, given a balanced diet. Creatine is believed to improve athletic performance, particularly explosive powerful exercise. If you wish to compete, creatine supplements may be something to consider taking before and after exercise. The dose is typically 0.1 gram of creatine per kilogram of body weight.

CURCUMIN. This powerful anti-inflammatory (found in the cooking spice turmeric) has been shown to alleviate and prevent symptoms of arthritis when taken in high concentrations. Curcurmin can also help alleviate joint soreness in the days following intense exercise. Ongoing research is exploring other possible health benefits, including chronic disease prevention. In general, curcumin reduces inflammation, and I prefer it to nonsteriodal anti-inflammatories (NSAIDs) such as aspirin or Aleve and Advil. Used to excess, NSAIDs can have a deleterious effect on your kidneys, liver, or stomach, depending on the particular formulation. Curcumin is often a better choice, though you won't get enough from adding spice to your food (you'd have to add so much that it would taste like dirt). A typical recommended dose is 300 milligrams twice daily. Be sure that the curcumin is in an active form, because it is a difficult supplement to source effectively.

DHEA. Think of dehydroepiandrosterone (DHEA) as a precursor to testosterone. If you recall from Chapter 4, DHEA is a prohormone secreted by the adrenal gland that is necessary to make testosterone. Supplementing with DHEA can help raise your testosterone levels and may prove especially useful as your hormonal levels, including DHEA, begin to decline in your thirties and forties. Folks with diabetes can be DHEA deficient, and some drugs, including insulin, interfere with the natural production of DHEA as well.

GLUCOSAMINE, CHONDROITIN, AND MSM. Joint products that combine these three supplements may help stimulate the production of healthy cartilage and improve the integrity of soft connective tissue. The bottom line is that you may feel less pain in joints and muscles, in addition to avoiding degenerative changes from arthritis over time.

GLUTAMINE. Glutamine is the most common amino acid found in your muscles. Exercise depletes these levels. Supplementing with glutamine will not only increase your lean muscle tissue, but also boost growth hormone levels and aid your immune system.

BETA-HYDROXY-BETA-METHYLBUTYRIC ACID (HMB). Found in grapefruit and catfish, HMB can be helpful in preventing muscle loss in the elderly, ill, and out of shape. Also, I find HMB useful in those recovering from an injury, or postoperative surgery on the shoulder, knee, or hip. It helps heal muscle faster.

MAGNESIUM. About half of your body's stores of magnesium are in the bones. They are also found in red blood cells. Magnesium is required for bone growth and is also believed to play a role in insulin regulation, as well as nerve and muscle function. In fact, it's the only mineral that crosses the blood-brain barrier, improving brain function. Found in most fiber-containing foods, such as leafy greens, legumes, and whole grain products, magnesium aids in digestion. It is also used in laxatives and antacids. If you exercise often and intensely, you may benefit from a magnesium supplement to increase energy and endurance.

OMEGA-3 FATTY ACIDS. The omega-3s, DHA and EPA, are involved in the metabolism of every cell in your body. They act as metabolic spark plugs that encourage fat loss; reduce risk for diabetes, heart disease, and stroke; fight inflammation; and offer brain-boosting benefits that may help prevent Alzheimer's disease. The American Heart Association recommends 4 grams of EPA and DHA per day, depending on your health risk. Be sure to check with your doctor if you take medications such as warfarin (Coumadin) or aspirin, as fish oils can thin your blood, too. When buying fish oil supplements, make sure the packaging says it is "pharmaceutical grade" oil. If you don't want the aftertaste of fish, you can look for an enteric-coated option, which will dissolve in your intestines rather than your stomach. Keeping this supplement in the refrigerator can also help to minimize the fishy reflux taste. Lovaza is a prescription version of omega fatty acids, as is Vascepta, a newly launched drug. Natural sources of omega-3s (and fiber) include flax-seeds, chia seeds, and hemp seeds. These little seeds help reduce your risk of heart disease, cancer, stroke, and diabetes. Flaxseeds and hemp seeds need to be ground just before use (coffee grinders work well) to make the nutrients available and to ensure the oils providing the omega-3s are fresh. Chia seeds can be used whole. Sprinkle ground hemp or flaxseed or whole chia seeds on your salads, into protein shakes, or on top of yogurt to fortify your meals with extra vitamins, minerals, healthy fats, and fiber.

OMEGA-6 FATTY ACIDS. These are often vilified in the media or even ignored due to their pervasiveness in the standard Western diet. Omega-6 fatty acids are needed for neural health and are available in supplement form, though you are likely getting enough through your diet. In Chapter 7, I mentioned that the ratio of omega-6s to omega-3s in an ideal diet should be 4–6 to 1, when really most Americans are getting anywhere from 6 to 10 times the amount of omega-6s we require. This disparity may be related to the spike in type 2 diabetes over the past few decades.

PROTEIN POWDERS. There is no shortage of protein options on the shelves of your local health food store. Whey protein isolate is the highest grade of whey protein currently available, and it is quickly and easily metabolized into your muscles. Whey is also a great source of branched chain amino acids, which are the building blocks of protein synthesis, your body's way of building muscle. The next best thing to whey is egg protein, otherwise known as casein. The biggest difference between whey and casein is that egg protein is absorbed into your body at a slower rate. This makes it a good option for breakfast if you do not work out in the morning, or at night if you eat an early dinner and get hungry later. Whey, on the other hand, is ideal for before or after your workout. There are plant-based protein powders for those looking for alternatives to dairy-based whey and casein. Gluten-free options are also available. Aim for protein powders with the fewest ingredients—preferably natural ingredients. If you want the most purity, there are flavorless protein powders whose only ingredient is whey protein isolate. Another option is protein bars, or snack bars with protein. Be forewarned: Numerous bars on the market include many processed ingredients you want to avoid. Aim for a bar containing 15 to 20 grams of protein and only natural ingredients. Again, the fewer ingredients, the better. There are bars out there to fit your vegan, kosher, dairy-free, and gluten-free requirements.

MULTIVITAMINS. Ideally, a daily multi may be insurance against any nutritional shortfalls you have in your diet. For some, a multi may be the best place to start. Which one you take depends on what is in the multi. Just watch out for iron. Unless you're deficient—your doctor can see this in your labs—adult men do not need to supplement iron. You are getting enough from what you are eating. Like I said earlier, I offer my patients FloQi Prime Power, which is a BioG MicroTab preparation that incorporates the multivitamin. Its benefits extend well beyond the generic multivitamin's indications with the addition of many supplements with universal benefits, such as emblica CoQ10, vitamin D, fruit and veggie powders, antioxidants, anti-inflammatories, and vitamins C and E.

RED YEAST RICE. Extracted from yeast that grows on rice, this supplement is a natural statin with cholesterol-lowering properties. It contains compounds called monacolins that can help inhibit cholesterol synthesis. All red yeast rices are not created equal; preparations have different degrees of activity and toxicity. Bottom line, red yeast rice can and often does play a role in reducing bad cholesterol. However, sourcing can determine how effective the supplement is. Remember, it is a drug and should be used only because you're trying to bring your cholesterol down. You'll know if it's working by the results of your follow-up blood tests. I have seen marked variations in response using red yeast rice from the same health food shop; response is not always predictable as the source and quality may not be the same.

SAW PALMETTO. Saw palmetto is a species of palm tree in the southeastern United States. Its fruit is used as the supplement. There is debate as to whether it can help the symptoms of an enlarged prostate by blocking a certain enzyme called 5 alpha-reductase. Acting like Propecia or Proscar, two brands of the generic drug finasteride, saw palmetto may also be used to prevent the conversion of testosterone to DHT and can remedy hair loss in some individuals. A newer to the market 5 alpha-reductase is dutasteride (Avodart). There is no generic version on the market as yet.

TESTOFEN. This is a supplement with multiple ingredients, including one called "mad goat weed." Data have shown that Testofen may have an effect on raising free testosterone.

ST. JOHN'S WORT. This supplement has been shown to help with mild symptoms of depression and sleep disorders. Ironically, using it in addition to antidepressants can hinder the effectiveness of an antidepressant. For many folks, it is a good addition to other treatments including exercise, diet, and medication. It is best to discuss with your personal physician to be sure that St. John's wort is safe to try.

Studies have been conducted to measure the effectiveness of this herb; however, as with all supplements, the source is crucial. Variables such as the soil, harvesting, storage, and manufacturing all impact the effectiveness of the herb. Be careful about buying any supplement that has no information on the label about quality control, bioactivity, and bioabsorption. Bioabsorption tells you whether or not the supplement will actually make it into your system at all.

———————————

This has been a brief listing of supplements. There are hundreds of options in your health food store, all of them promising different benefits. Remember to do your research—there are great manufacturers out there, as well as products that consist of nothing more than sugar powder at best and, at worst, dangerous toxins. Work with your doctor to make smart supplement choices and use your personal health metrics to guide you.

CHAPTER 9

THE TRUTH ABOUT HORMONE THERAPIES

Check your levels and then consider your options

You now know you will go through andropause just like women go through menopause. You also know it's going to be a gradual process. After your mid- to late twenties, testosterone begins to decline by roughly 1 to 3 percent a year, accelerating as you age. Remember, this happens because the brain stops playing along as it should. Instead of using LH (luteinizing hormone) and GnRH (gonadotropin-releasing hormone) to stimulate the testes to produce more testosterone, the brain begins to adjust to the new lower levels. Testosterone continues to drop off, with free circulating T often well below what's needed to maintain peak metabolic function. Remember that free T is usable T. It represents the amount of testosterone that is circulating and able to bind to receptor sites. In general, I like to see free T between

150 and 200 picograms per deciliter (pg/dL), whereas total T should be between 800 and 1200 pg/dL for optimal function. Remember, though, these are just ranges, and I focus on what's best for you. Lifestyle, genetics, illness, and personal factors all play a part as well.

An option when you have low testosterone is to optimize your levels with therapies including testosterone and hCG. Here's how they can help:

- **You will have more energy.** Testosterone will give you more energy to move. Exercise is also a terrific natural antidepressant, and you'll be able to do more of it with less fatigue. Your psychological outlook becomes more positive, especially as you see results.

- **You will produce muscle.** Testosterone is one of the basic building blocks of muscle. You'll likely notice gains as your testosterone increases. The ability to produce muscle means your time spent working out will be more efficient, plus recovery will be quicker.

- **Your metabolism will rise.** Your testosterone rises because you're building more muscle. Muscle itself is active tissue and will help your body burn calories after the workout and even at rest.

- **Your athletic performance will improve.** This is an unmistakable outcome to muscle production and more intense workouts. But more to the point, you'll *want* to play more golf or soccer or basketball, whatever your game is.

- **You will feel stronger.** You will have more stamina and feel younger.

- **Your health will change for the better.** You will lose weight and redistribute muscle and fat to healthier proportions on your body (body composition tests confirm this, as does tightening your belt around a leaner midsection). What's more, your body will respond in other positive ways. Blood pressure and resting heart rate may improve. Cholesterol ratios and triglyceride measurements often improve as well. Your immune system may become more effective, freeing up some of those sick days for vacation time.

- **Your body will metabolize sugar better.** Your weight loss, associated with testosterone treatment, may reverse insulin resistance, metabolic syndrome, and even diabetes.

- **You will feel more confident.** Your brain fog will clear and your mood may improve.

- **Your sex drive will return.** Testosterone will help fuel this, and so will all the other gains I just mentioned.

COMING OUT OF THE SHADOWS ... TESTOSTERONE OPTIMIZATION

Testosterone treatment is probably familiar to you. And maybe not in a good way. About 40 percent of my patients are doctors, yet sometimes they are resistant to hormone therapy because of the distorted stories in the press about testosterone and steroid abuse among athletes and, bodybuilders. Also, endocrinology is a select specialty of medicine. Most doctors don't receive adequate training in hormone physiology and, therefore, are not familiar with using testosterone, estrogen, or supplements like DHEA. Endocrinologists who treat adults mostly focus on diabetes, as well as thyroid and bone disease, along with other types of endocrine disorders. Urologists are also specialists who tend to focus on prostate and bladder function, typically paying less attention to hormones. More specific to men, there are doctors who treat male infertility—men with underactive testes, who may not make enough sperm, or men with anatomical abnormalities such as varicocele. That field differs from andrology, which is the study of male hormone function. Andrology, as I mentioned in the beginning of the book, actually does not exist as a formal field of medical practice.

Likely the most pervasive, incorrect assumption about treating patients with testosterone is that it causes prostate cancer. This is not true. In fact, prostate cancer risk actually rises as testosterone levels fall with age, making it harder to reconcile the cause and effect relationship between testosterone treatment and cancer. Second, causation is extremely difficult to determine in medicine given each person's individual makeup and history. And remember, to establish significance with a good deal of validity, studies need to be extremely well controlled and sample sizes need to be large, often amassing a group that's as homogenous as possible. The fact is, the study upon which this testosterone-prostate cancer link is based was done on just 13 men (yes, *13*) in the 1930s (or around 80 years ago). These men, who all had low testosterone and untreated prostate cancer, already metastatic, were randomly treated with or without testosterone. Those treated with testosterone died a few years prior to those who were not. Despite its small sample size and datedness, this study has completely skewed the field of hormone therapy for decades and unfoundedly frightened a lot of people.

In a study published in 2004 in the *New England Journal of Medicine*, Abraham Morgentaler, MD, an associate clinical professor of urology at Harvard Medical School, found no evidence that men with higher testosterone levels were at greater risk of prostate cancer. In fact, Dr. Morgentaler confirms in his book *Testosterone for Life*, "new evidence shows that low T, rather than high T, may be a risk for prostate cancer." Since then there have been more than a dozen longitudinal studies examining the relationship between hormones and prostate cancer, and not one has shown a direct correlation between the level of total testosterone in a man's blood and the likelihood that he will develop prostate cancer. As of this writing, the science shows that even when you put a group of men with early prostate cancer on testosterone and you conduct second biopsies following T treatment, there is no change in the cancerous cells—testosterone doesn't make them grow or proliferate.

One of my patients with early-stage prostate cancer goes to see another doctor at an academic center in New York who is an expert in prostate cancer. Upon hearing about my patient's interest in beginning testosterone treatment, the doctor was in agreement because it would help turn around the patient's underlying cardiac disease and diabetes, both of which posed more immediate harm to his health than the prostate cancer. The doctor performed follow-up biopsies on my patient 1 and 2 years after he started testosterone therapy, and there was no further growth of the prostate cancer. He was monitored by "active surveillance." Meanwhile, the testosterone was helping to reverse his other medical problems.

It is important to note that while testosterone does not cause prostate cancer, it may bring an underlying, undetected cancer to light. Testosterone stimulates the prostate, and PSA levels may rise as a result. A PSA level above 4 ng/mL will likely warrant further attention. It is important to watch for benign prostatic hyperplasia (BPH), which may result from elevated PSA levels if too much testosterone is being converted to DHT. However, if you are taking finasteride (Proscar) or dutasteride (Avodart) to block the conversion of T to DHT and your PSA is still increasing, then you may need to consult with your doctor. She may want to measure your percent free PSA, which I'll discuss in Chapter 10.

I find it interesting that little attention is paid to the role played by suboptimal levels of testosterone in the increase of disease and the shortening of life span. Yet there are articles that have shown such relationships do exist; that is, the lower the testosterone, the earlier morbidity and mortality in men. Meanwhile, estrogen's part in the emergence of disease in women gets tons of press.

Hormone therapy became a popular treatment option for women partly because it is so easy to determine when it might be needed. Menopause begins with clear physical signs like hot flashes and irregular periods, all leading up to the cessation of menstruation. As women experience these hormonal changes, they feared they would look and feel old (on top of sensing a profound shift in their role in society). What I see in clinical practice when I use hormone therapy, however, is that women's response takes time and, because their cycles are often unpredictable, it's difficult to gauge their progress and response. Conversely, men's response to hormone therapy is more rapid and they see a corresponding uptick in sexual function, libido, energy, and more in a matter of weeks.

Despite the evidence, very little attention has been given to testosterone's role in the aging process for men, and also for women.

Part of the problem is that treatment with testosterone has just recently been brought to the attention of physicians, ironically due to commercials touting the benefits of T. Yet public media focuses on the abuse of steroids by professional athletes, which overshadows the effect of testosterone seen in clinical practice. Meanwhile, the data on testosterone and its positive effect on various organ systems has been published across multiple disciplines—cardiology, urology, psychology, and others—over the past couple of decades. Still, many doctors (and regular folks) do feel that aging is "natural," so why intervene? Most doctors are not inclined to introduce controversial therapies into their practices, and for good reason. Little incentive exists to pursue testosterone's use clinically, and this is driven by a lack of understanding, and maybe time, as well as a neglect for the aspects of aging that could be averted.

What's more, some of this research involves older men well past the thirties/forties benchmark when testosterone levels begin declining. In one study, testosterone therapy was halted after several men had heart attacks and cardiovascular events. The results were still published in the *New England Journal of Medicine*; however, the investigators noted their research's limitations, specifically, the age of the men being studied—all older, over 65. Another study found that men (again, 65 plus) with naturally high levels of testosterone had higher cardiovascular risk than those with lower levels. Increased cardiovascular risk has been documented in the literature for women receiving estrogen replacement therapy as well. Studies showed an increase in breast cancer and heart disease after 5 years of oral treatment. But estrogen or progesterone pills are often synthetic derivatives, and the patients were also generally older and not screened for preexisting conditions.

In the fall of 2012, JoAnn Manson, a professor of medicine at Harvard Medical School and Brigham and Women's Hospital, presented findings from her KEEPS trial. These showed that hormone treatment, both oral and transdermal, had many positive effects in *newly* postmenopausal women with an average age of 52.7 years. In fact, certain findings, like one that stated that estrogen treatment has no negative effect on cognitive function, ran counter to research done by the Women's Health Initiative of the NIH on postmenopausal women age 65 and older.

Many times, the patients recruited for these studies do not receive thorough evaluations before they start treatment (or, in some cases, receive a placebo, if the study is a double-blind randomized controlled trial). Chronic disease may be the cause of adverse events, not the testosterone or estrogen. Because of the timing, however, it's assumed to be directly related to the treatment. The same is likely true of the older men in the *New England Journal of Medicine* study I just spoke about. Patients who are not screened for preexisting conditions may have an underlying disease. If they become symptomatic during the study, it is not clear that testosterone or any other hormone causes the emergence of that disease. I know this is a complicated concept; however, it speaks to the challenges faced by doctors who want to interpret the studies yet are stymied by the outcomes and how to apply the data. Above all, we take an oath to "do no harm," and the risks to patients experimenting with any new or untested treatment are understandable and shouldn't be taken lightly. All I'm suggesting is that sometimes our fear of not knowing inhibits our willingness to explore further.

What's more, the abuses we hear about in the media involve testosterone or other androgen steroids being used in megadoses, 10 to 100 times physiological levels, which will throw the body completely out of balance. At the center of these stories are often younger men whose bodies are still able to produce their own testosterone. In flooding their systems with exogenous testosterone, they're effectively halting their body's natural production of testosterone. Often, the consequences of this sort of inappropriate overuse are grave. There are physical symptoms like testicular shrinkage and additional breast tissue, and years down the line the body may not show an adequate response to treatment with either testosterone or hCG (human chorionic gonadotropin). One of my patients is in his midtwenties with a history of testosterone abuse. When I started him on hormone injections to get his body to produce its own testosterone once again, his response was sluggish. It took longer for him to react than it did for most men who are new to hormone treatment.

I only prescribe what will work best for each patient. Some patients don't require any hormonal intervention. Some require more than others. Whatever you use, it has to be appropriate to balance your body. You or your doctor won't know whether you need hormone therapy until the lab data comes back and all your clinical findings are analyzed. Additionally, as with any medical intervention, you should also take into account your personal and family history as well as lifestyle choices.

METHOD OF DELIVERY AND STARTING TREATMENT

When I treat women with estrogen, I prescribe estrogen in a topical form. Hormone replacement therapy, popularized in the 1980s, primarily used oral estrogen, which was extracted from the urine of pregnant mares. My feeling is that, in general, the pill caused more harm than good. I never prescribed oral Premarin, even when it was popular. It's an estrogen that has been shown to increase risk for breast cancer and heart disease. It also has to travel through the liver, which increases cholesterol. Even 25 years ago, I used a women's health pharmacy that compounded bioidentical estrogen and testosterone creams. "Bioidentical" means that these hormones were derived from plants and synthesized in a lab to have the exact same structure and functionality as actual hormones. Today, bioidentical hormones are gaining popularity, yet they were unique at the time.

For men, testosterone delivered either orally or topically is *not preferable*, in my opinion. Oral testosterone, like oral estrogen, has to go through the liver, which again has a negative effect on cholesterol. In fact, in the United States, oral testosterone is almost never prescribed due to these side effects. Buccal (under the tongue) testosterone may bypass the liver but can be erratic. With topical treatment, attaining appropriate levels is challenging. What's more, cream or gels can be transferred through skin-to-skin contact, and testosterone given to men is in a dosage that's dangerous to women and children. Men who use this form of testosterone may also suffer from unwanted side effects. Because body fat is rich in the enzyme aromatase, when a man uses a topical cream or gel, testosterone will come in contact with the aromatase as the hormone is absorbed. If you recall from Chapter 4, this interaction—aromatase meets testosterone—produces estrogen in the form of estradiol in an amount that is too high for a man. Another enzyme, 5-alpha reductase, is also present in skin: When it comes in contact with topical testosterone, the body will make more dihydrotestosterone (DHT), possibly causing hair loss and enlargement of the prostate gland (not cancerous).

Testosterone injections, on the other hand, bypass these enzymes in the skin as well as the liver. In general, injected T produces a stronger physiological effect than the oral or topical methods of delivery. Most of the men I see inject 50 to 200 milligrams (0.25 to 1.0 cubic centimeters) every week. Some men require injections twice a week due to more rapid metabolism, while others inject at 2-week intervals. You use a small needle to inject subcutaneously, meaning under the skin as opposed to intramuscularly. Injectable forms of T use oil as the transfer agent, which makes the solution viscous, requiring you to inject more slowly with a thinner needle.

When testosterone levels rise with treatment, so too do the number of red blood cells, as red blood cells carry oxygen. This means more oxygen is available throughout the body (the Lance Armstrong effect!), which is helpful when you are active at higher altitudes. Once you begin optimizing your testosterone, a doctor should monitor your labs to watch out for a high red blood cell count that can make your bloodflow sluggish. If your red blood cell count is too high, you can donate a unit of blood.

Note: Testosterone therapy may affect fertility, because therapy essentially takes over the testes' job of producing testosterone. This is why I generally only prescribe testosterone to men who are going through andropause or are already beyond it. The testes' response at this point is diminished, and the body is unable to produce enough testosterone on its own. As a result, fertility suffers. While the man's sperm may still be viable at this point in his life, the sperm can change in their nature or movement—for instance, there may be fewer of them (less than 20 million sperm per cubic centimeter), they may be less motile, or abnormal in appearance. If you are someone who may benefit from testosterone ther-

Options for Testosterone Optimization

I treat patients who have low T primarily with injectable hCG or testosterone. There are other therapies that may be more feasible for you to use. Before beginning testosterone, you should have your baseline lab data analyzed by a trained physician who can monitor your progress. Tell your doctor how you're feeling upon beginning treatment. Your self-report is actually more relevant than your lab numbers. The treatment options:

HCG injections. Human chorionic gonadotropin (hCG) is not testosterone but rather a natural protein hormone purified from the urine of pregnant women. It mimics luteinizing hormone (LH) to stimulate the testes to produce testosterone. Whenever possible I like to help the body do what it does naturally. Compounded by a pharmaceutical company, it is reconstituted with sterile water and injected into the abdomen by the patient twice weekly. I use hCG often in patients who have not yet hit andropause, meaning both their testosterone and LH are low. *Brand name:* Pregnyl and Novarel. *Generic:* hCG, and Compound versions. *Downside:* Not for the needle-phobic, though the needle is tiny and barely felt; expensive unless compounded version is utilized. Speak to your physician.

Intramuscular or subcutaneous injection. Testosterone is injected with a syringe into the thigh or buttocks by a physician weekly, but it's more convenient to DIY at home. There are thinner subcutaneous gauge needles that you can use that cause less pain. Once a man undergoes andropause, I usually recommend that he switch from using hCG to injectable testosterone. Sometimes I cycle between the two (example: T for 10 weeks, then hCG for 4) before transitioning to testosterone. The lab data helps to signify when a man has entered andropause—often LH will rise while testosterone remains low. *Brand name:* Depo-testosterone. *Generic:* Cypionate and Enanthate. *Downside:* Inconvenient; not for the needle-phobic, though the subcutaneous route is tolerable.

Mouth patch. A tablet placed next to the upper gums twice a day delivers testosterone continuously into the bloodstream bypassing the stomach and avoiding potential liver toxicity. *Brand name:* Striant. *Downside:* Inconvenient, can cause gum irritation, uneven levels.

apy and are considering possible pregnancy with a partner during treatment, you should have a semen count before beginning therapy. You may want to schedule a consultation with a fertility expert. Another alternative is to use hCG instead of testosterone.

Subcutaneous implant. Small pellets about the size of a grain of rice are implanted through a 1-inch incision in the buttocks or abdomen and replaced every 3 to 6 months. *Brand name:* Testopel. *Downside:* Quarterly doctor visits; expensive.

Topical gel. Available in packets or pumps, the clear testosterone gel is applied once a day to the shoulders and upper arms. *Brand name:* AndroGel, Testim and Fortesta. Axiron is applied like deodorant to the underarms. *Downside:* Can be inadvertently transferred to women and children through touch with serious side effects.

Transdermal patch. A medicine-coated skin patch applied once a day to the upper arm, upper body or scrotum supplies a steady dose of testosterone. *Brand name:* Androderm and Testoderm. *Downside:* Can cause skin irritation, inconvenient.

Testosterone Supplement. Available without a prescription, this supplement contains Fenugreek extract. Data has shown this extract helps raise free testosterone. *Brand name:* Testofen. *Downside:* Dietary supplements are not regulated by the FDA, so purity and efficacy cannot be guaranteed.

Oral testosterone pills. These are almost never prescribed in the US because of the risk of liver toxicity and negative effects on cholesterol. Pharmaceutical companies are testing a soft capsule form of testosterone undecanoate that is supposed to foster absorption in the intestine and protect the liver.

ON THE HORIZON: **Long-acting testosterone undecanoate.** A testosterone formulation that is injected about every 10 weeks, offering greater convenience, is available in more than 90 countries. Concerns about microembolism to the lungs have prevented the drug from being brought to the US marketplace. *Brand name:* Aveed. *Downside:* Potential microembolism to the lungs.

PREANDROPAUSE? HCG MAY JUMP-START YOUR SYSTEM

The human body is an elegant and complex system. My preference is to support the system to operate at its best as opposed to replacing or suppressing a function using a drug to stand in for something that's naturally occurring in the body. That's why I use the hormone hCG—it helps the body to help itself. Whenever possible, I believe it's best to have the body produce its own hormones, to establish its own equilibrium. Under the right circumstances, hCG will trigger the testes to generate testosterone, thus mimicking the natural process and acting as LH.

As you'll recall, human chorionic gonadotropin is a natural hormone distilled from the urine of pregnant women. When a woman conceives, hCG is produced by the placenta and is critical for a healthy pregnancy. Pregnancy tests typically measure rising levels of hCG, and hCG is also commonly used in fertility centers. When a couple undergoes in vitro fertilization, hCG is the hormone given via intramuscular injection in the woman, critically timed to release multiple eggs from her ovaries, resulting in ovulation.

My background work in fertility, puberty, and reproductive function led me to choose hCG as my preferred starting point for optimizing testosterone in men. In my clinical research, I had worked with the brain hormone, gonadotropin-releasing hormone (GnRH), to reverse teenage development in young children with precocious puberty and to induce puberty in others with delayed onset of adulthood. (Research has also been done on using hCG to stimulate puberty in young men who are lacking the hormones to trigger development.) My understanding of the communication loop between the brain and the hormones of the sex organs helped me to recognize the potential benefit of hCG. It acts on this same loop. Having spent decades exploring new therapeutic interventions in clinical research with many NIH protocols and FDA investigational drug studies, I was comfortable with alternate, off-label uses of medication.

Hormone Use in the World of Professional Sports

In 2009, the Cleveland Indians suspended Manny Ramirez for testing positive for hCG during spring training that year. It cost the outfielder 50 games on the bench. Some speculated that he was taking hCG to mask a course of steroids or mitigate its symptoms, such as testicular shrinkage and low sperm count. He may have taken it to help restart his body's own production of testosterone if he indeed was on steroids. Others deemed his hCG use legitimate, because the hormone has been shown to help male infertility and raise testosterone levels. I don't know why Ramirez chose to use hCG or if he actually did; however, let's consider his age at the time of the controversy—37. It is highly plausible that his body was already beginning its decline, his testosterone dropping each year. The question I have then is: Why shouldn't we help him stay at his peak with hCG in combination with other medications, supplements, and lifestyle decisions, these proactive choices benefiting both his athletic performance and, more important, his overall health?

I encourage all men to get blood work in their twenties so that they have a baseline and know their hormone levels at their physiologic and reproductive peak. As long as levels are monitored closely by a medical professional and hCG isn't abused, there could be a fair avenue to lengthen not only careers but also performance in athletes. Then a player in his thirties or forties could legally use performance enhancers, which would actually be seen as performance *retainers* at that point, because there would be essentially no change in their testosterone levels as compared to when they were in their twenties. We could then define "abuse" or "performance enhancement" as a player being above the reference range for too long. Another option would be to just play it safe and use very small doses of things like hCG and testosterone when initiating treatment. Obviously, the governing bodies in sports will have to determine where they want to go. I would hope that a serious look, not just for enhanced performance but for life and health, is debated and discussed, given testosterone's impact on body and mind. These athletes are paid millions: Why not put some of that money toward understanding longevity and well-being? Maybe that will help all of us, including you.

A very small number of doctors prescribe hCG as a fertility treatment, and even fewer prescribe it to stimulate testosterone production and increase health span. Because this therapy has not yet become mainstream, getting a prescription may be difficult. Only an experienced physician should recommend hCG, which is prescribed as a powder and needs to be mixed with sterile water (it also comes premixed). Typically, you inject between 1,000 milli-international units (mIU) and 5,000 mIU twice per week. Your doctor should monitor your blood levels of testosterone—as well as other hormones and metabolites that may be produced—through routine tests that ideally occur after 3 months, then at longer intervals, such as two or three times annually. That way, the dosage and injection frequency can be adjusted as needed. Initially, I prefer to test after 4 to 6 weeks and adjust according to the hormone levels reflected in lab data as well as the effect my patient reports clinically. That is: How is he feeling overall? In my experience, most men typically feel different within weeks, and after the first couple of months on hCG, I usually monitor them less frequently. The main aim is to provide a physiological balance that allows your body to function optimally and maintains your sense of well-being naturally.

FAQS ABOUT HCG?

1. WHAT IS THE HCG DIET? A fraudulent version of hCG called "homeopathic hCG" has recently been banned by the Food and Drug Administration. These homeopathic oral drops, unverified by mainstream science, are popular among those who ascribe to the hCG diet, where hCG is administered in combination with a strict and quite dangerous starvation diet of just 500 calories a day. Of course you will lose weight by consuming only 500 calories. You will also lose lean muscle and will become malnourished. Once you begin to consume more calories, your weight rebound may be significant. The diet really has nothing to do with hCG. What's more, these homeopathic hCG drops or pills will be digested and unlikely to be absorbed—never the best for efficacy when it comes to hormones—so they will not have an appreciable effect on your body.

2. WHAT IS THE DIFFERENCE BETWEEN HCG AND HGH? It may be because the acronyms hCG and HGH are similar and that both have been implicated in high-profile sports controversies, but I hear a lot of confusion—people seem to think HGH and hCG are one and the same. You'll recall from Chapter 4 that human growth hormone (HGH) is produced by the brain's pituitary gland to spur growth in children. As adults, HGH continues to maintain the health of organs and tissues, though we produce less of it. Growth hormone is released during sleep, which is one reason sleep is so crucial. How much HGH levels drop with age and how consistently the decline happens is not as predictable as the falloff in testosterone, which ultimately and steadily drops in men (and women) over the course of time. Since I can't measure HGH, I rely on IGF-1 to tell me if there is a cause for concern. I prescribe HGH much less frequently than testosterone or hCG. I only write a script if IGF-1 levels if a man's labs are very low, typically less than 100 to 150 ng/mL after 6 to 12 months on L-arginine and citrulline supplementation, with improvements in exercise and sleep, evidence of elevated testosterone, and an increase in lean muscle. Another reason I would give HGH injections might be the presence of poor carbohydrate metabolism (indicated by an elevated fasting glucose, fasting insulin, and/or high hemoglobin A1c) combined with low IGF-1. This is because there is data suggesting that too little HGH contributes to diabetes and obesity.

3. WHAT DO YOU DO WHEN HGC STOPS WORKING? Even given injections of prescription hCG, at some point a man's testicles will stop responding to the hormone. Testosterone levels will begin to once again decline. Treatment with hCG is not a permanent solution, and your body will continue to mature and age naturally while you're using the hormone hCG. When that onset of andropause begins, I often switch men to testosterone. A lot of men ask me if using hCG will cause their testes to stop responding, moving their systems into andropause earlier than might be expected had they not received treatment. To my knowledge, hCG does not hasten andropause, and the testes will continue to produce their own testosterone naturally for as long as they can. This can be years—I've had patients produce their own testosterone into their eighties. That's not common, however. I usually see the testes' function petering out in the fifties and sixties; again, though, this cutoff varies from man to man. The transition to andropause in men can last for decades—unlike women, where the average menopausal age is 51.8 years and the window of time when menopause occurs is narrower. Often, as a man moves through andropause, I cycle hCG and testosterone treatment until the response to hCG is negligible. For instance, I may prescribe 4 weeks of hCG followed by 10 weeks of T.

Critics argue that there are no legitimate long-term studies of this kind of hCG use. They are right. One study published in the *Journal of Clinical Endocrinology and Metabolism* found that 3 months of twice-weekly hCG treatment did indeed raise testosterone and muscle mass, yet had no effect on muscle strength and physical functioning. Understand, however, this study was simply a measure of how hCG affects the body *without* a nutrition and fitness component. Even more important, it was a short-term pilot trial, only 3 months, which was limiting in that the researchers were unable to measure hCG's effect over a longer period of time. Eat right and exercise with hCG, as my patients do, and everything acts in concert. That increase in testosterone goes to work producing lean muscle mass, and helping your metabolism function better. Men's lives have been transformed by this therapy. In research circles, the proof I've seen in my clinical practice is considered anecdotal evidence and isn't taken as seriously as long-term, peer-reviewed research published in highly regarded journals. Publishing the data I have collected would be ideal, and I plan to do so. My initial abstract describes this decline in testosterone associated with lack of response of the brain hormones, using scientific speak to describe the baseball analogy I laid out in Chapter 1. *Hormonal Expression of Androgen Decline in Aging Men*, the title of our research data, was presented at the Endocrine Society meeting in San Francisco on June 15, 2013, and our article is pending review.

I've been challenged to justify my approach at every turn in my medical career. Once, when I was a junior faculty member at Yale, a very well respected doctor and department head said to me, "The problem with you, Florence, is that you're an independent thinker."

He didn't mean it as a compliment. But I took it as one.

I was reading a lot online about hCG as a way to stimulate T, when I had my own hormonal levels drawn. I found out my T was on the low side, and so I got hCG and I started treating myself. It was 500 units, three times a week.

So, first of all: Why was I doing this? I was feeling kind of lethargic. My mood was low. I didn't have clinical depression. I had a lack of energy. All of us tend to struggle a little bit with weight or body fat percentage. That's normal. I am running a very busy cosmetic practice, 60 to 70 hours a week. It was not that I wasn't functioning, but it's just that I felt blah.

Trying hCG myself wasn't necessarily experimental. There's nothing unusual about the use of hCG. I just wanted to decide first if I thought it worked. When I began taking hCG, I noticed my mood was a little elevated. When I redrew my levels, there were some improvements. I did enough of it to believe that it worked, after which I said to myself: What the hell are you doing? This really isn't your specialty. Why don't you get some-one to monitor you and optimize you? I came across Florence's information and I read the article "Vigor Quest" in the *New York Times*. The reason I chose Florence was her background in reproductive endocrinology. Her qualifications for age manage-ment are really ideal.

Taken together, Florence's program gave me a youthfulness, but vigor even more than youthfulness. I've worked out before; I still work out. My workouts are more productive. I've got more muscle mass. Of all the improvements, the best one is probably in my head, meaning my mood. And I think that comes back to testosterone more than anything. I would be less than candid with you if I didn't say that I think it's 70 percent hormonal manipulation.

—MICHAEL R., MD, age 56, surgeon

Hormones are not the only answer; however, they can help move your body into that sweet spot so that it's primed for change. To take advantage of that opportunity, you will have to make the personal investment I've outlined in Chapters 5 to 7. In the next chapter, you'll learn about advanced testing that may be warranted given the results of your lab data. These tests will give your doctor more specific information about what your needs are and how your body responds to medications and supplements.

CHAPTER **10**

ADVANCED DIAGNOSTICS
More tests for maximizing your health span

E verything you've read in this book has been about achieving one goal: maximizing your health span. Your personal health metrics taken together with your lab data have indicated the issues for you to prioritize. If you have begun to make lifestyle changes and added a highly personalized cocktail of supplements, maybe even started the process to optimize your testosterone, you are on your way to enjoying a good quality of life as you age.

Your health, like everything else in life, is an ongoing journey. The next step in the process is one that's more finely tuned and won't be applicable for everybody. Advanced diagnostic testing will help you learn even more about who you are and what you might expect in your future. Many physicians would consider these evaluations radical, and argue that they are unnecessary and cost too much. They generally won't order these tests until you show symptoms of a disease. Sounds like a valid point of view, right? Does it really make sense to undergo an investigative process at such an early stage? Why not wait? I see this perspective as *disease* care, not health care. Diseases can take a toll quickly and appear suddenly. Once they manifest, reversal is less likely, the cost of management more, the quality of life diminished. I want to preserve my health, and the health of my patients.

These tests will help you maximize your lifestyle choices and interventional options to make them even more personalized for you. For instance, your doctor may want to put you on a statin for your high cholesterol. Getting particle testing done by Berkeley HeartLab, however, may reveal that even though your LDL is high, you actually may not need a statin. You see not all LDL particles are created equal. The larger, fluffy LDL particles are cardioprotective, while the smaller, sticky ones can cause disease.

Although there are many possible ways to look at advanced testing, this chapter focuses on descriptions of follow-up tests for carbohydrate metabolism, cardiopulmonary health, lipid metabolism, and thyroid issues. It discusses advanced imaging, highly individualized blood tests, and genetic DNA analyses. Quite often, obtaining an answer from your blood work or another assessment leads to new questions pertaining to your diagnosis or treatment options. This is a good thing. More specific questions often leads to finding the right answer.

CARB METABOLISM

GLUCOSE TOLERANCE TEST

This lab test checks how your body handles and breaks down sugar over 2 to 4 hours. This would be an advanced diagnostic test if your baseline lab tests suggest a risk of diabetes based on your fasting sugar, insulin, and/or your hemoglobin A1c. If these three measures are not in the acceptable reference range, and particularly if you have a family history of diabetes, this test would be helpful to sort out what is going on in your body with respect to sugar metabolism. My recommendation is that it be done if your fasting blood sugar is over 94 mg/dL, your fasting insulin is over 5 mcIU/mL, and/or your hemoglobin A1c is 5.7 percent or higher. Family history and other risk factors, such as weakness or feeling shaky or dizzy 2 to 3 hours after eating, would contribute to determining if this test might be useful for you. How you do on this test will help you further customize your program for sleep (8 hours helps maintain insulin levels), food (protein, fiber, and frequent small meals stabilize blood sugar), and fitness. (Interval training can help, even if you are a type 1 diabetic. Monitor your sugar levels more closely and ingest an appropriate snack before and after exercise.) The results will also shape your future monitoring as well as the proper interventions.

The most common glucose tolerance test is the *oral glucose tolerance test* (OGTT, also GTT). Before the test begins, a sample of blood will be drawn. You'll be asked to drink a liquid containing a certain amount of glucose, usually 75 grams, on an empty stomach. To measure your glucose and insulin levels at each checkpoint, your blood will be taken again every 30 to 60 minutes after you drink the solution.

The test takes up to 2 to 4 hours. I typically perform a 2-hour OGTT, though selectively a 3-hour OGTT makes sense depending on symptoms (for example, feeling weak or shaky). To prepare for the OGTT, make sure you eat normally for several days prior to the test. You must fast, for at least 8 to 12 hours before the test. (You are allowed to drink water.) Ask your doctor if any medications or supplements could affect results. Some people feel nauseated, sweaty, or lightheaded. They sometimes become short of breath or faint after drinking the glucose. It is unlikely for most people to have any serious side effects though.

Lately, I was always feeling sick. My job was high stress, though I was always told that my performance was outstanding. I recently retired, partly because I was working 24/7, always on the road, and having trouble making it through the day. Sleep was always fragmented. I would feel weak and fatigued within 2 to 3 hours after eating and would have to lie down. The kind of work I did just didn't allow for that possibility.

I guess I was what you might call one of those high-powered executive salesman types. I was in meetings all day, and I would count on my bagel and OJ after my morning workouts to hold me through until a client dinner, which was almost always at a steak house. By then I'd have the 12-ounce filet and the baked potato and the creamed corn and dessert because I was real hungry. For a while, I was okay living this way. It wasn't ideal, but it was what I felt I had to do, you know?

Dr. Comite and her team had told me I was a prediabetic. My hemoglobin A1c was 5.7, and she recommended more regular snacks with more protein, especially at the start of my day. I appreciated what she was saying, but I never really took action because she said I was borderline. In other words, I didn't think things were that bad.

Eventually though, I started feeling really crappy by 11:00 a.m. Going 4 to 5 hours, or even only 2 or 3, without eating wasn't working anymore. At that point, I called Dr. Comite, and she sent me in for a glucose tolerance test. Sure enough, the test confirmed that I had reactive hypoglycemia. Because I was on my way to becoming a diabetic, everyone had thought my blood sugar would be too high, not too low. No one had suspected hypoglycemia, and I certainly was never tested. Now that I've retired, I've changed my lifestyle completely. I'm conscious of what I eat and when I eat. It's kind of amazing that the more successful you become, the unhealthier you can actually get. I guess it means you just have to work that much harder. But the payoff—having energy and not feeling like hell—it's worth it.

—SAM P., age 62, retired vice president of sales

Normal blood values for a 75-gram oral glucose tolerance test used to check for type 2 diabetes:

- Fasting: 60 to 95 milligrams per deciliter (mg/dL). My optimal target range would be 60 to 85 mg/dL.
- 1 hour: less than 200 mg/dL

- 2 hours: less than 140 mg/dL. Optimal would be less than 100 mg/dL, or even reaching the fasting range. (Optimal value ranges may vary slightly among different laboratories because they have slightly varying assays.)

Higher than acceptable levels of glucose may be indicative of diabetes. Levels between 100 and 200 mg/dL is called impaired glucose tolerance and signifies a disorder of carbohydrate metabolism. Your doctor may call this prediabetes, meaning you are at increased risk for developing diabetes. A glucose level of 200 mg/dL or higher is a sign of diabetes. Rarely, high glucose levels may be related to another medical problem—for example, Cushing's syndrome, which is an overproduction of cortisol, the stress hormone. A higher than acceptable insulin level is also abnormal and points to insulin resistance. Lower than acceptable glucose levels suggest hypoglycemia, which may be a prelude to diabetes. Once again the point is, one sign does not necessarily indicate a direct relationship between symptom and disease. Talk to your doctor about the meaning of your specific test results, especially if you have identified other risk modifiers.

CARDIOPULMONARY HEALTH

CARDIAC STRESS TEST

Stress tests have been done by cardiologists for decades, either via echocardiogram (sonogram) or nuclear scan. An echocardiogram is frequently and simply referred to as an "echo." It will show the valves (the connectors between chambers of the heart and from the heart to the lungs or body). It will check for abnormal leakage creating murmurs that your doctor might hear on an exam with her stethoscope. Visualization during a stress test will reveal your heart muscle motion. A nuclear scan identifies damaged heart muscle and tells me how well your heart is pumping blood. Still, sufficient disease has to be present in order to detect a problem. If results of a stress test show abnormalities, an immediate investigation is launched, potentially requiring an angiogram with angioplasty and/or the placement of stents, or even open heart surgery. At times, there are false positives, meaning the test is abnormal though the heart vessels are fine. A positive test is usually followed by a cardiac catheterization (done in a specialized lab usually in a hospital) to detect if there are significant blockages in your coronary arteries. On rare occasions, false negative tests also happen and may unfortunately not detect cardiac disease that can lead to a heart attack.

VO$_2$ ASSESSMENT

Beyond the stress test, the VO$_2$ assessment allows a more specific understanding of how your heart, lungs, and skeletal muscles are functioning. It measures your maximum oxygen consumption while you exercise on a treadmill or a bike. The work rate increases over time. The assessment lasts approximately 10 minutes, where you'll engage both your aerobic and anaerobic systems, moving from one to the other over the course of the test. The VO$_2$ assessment is the gold standard for measuring your level of physical fitness. Improvements in VO$_2$ score point to increased fat utilization and overall gains in cardiopulmonary performance. Average scores vary with age, gender, and altitude, and sometimes a poor VO$_2$ score is surprising, telling even. As I mentioned in Chapter 7, Livingston Miller's VO$_2$ score was alarmingly low, especially in light of his degree of fitness. Essentially, a man at his age who's healthy and at his level of training should have had a VO$_2$ score of around 50 mL/kg/min, and his was hovering somewhere around 20 mL/kg/min. His heart wasn't able to perform adequately, and I immediately referred him for further testing. He underwent a nuclear stress test, which unfortunately confirmed that he had experienced a "silent" myocardial infarction (a heart attack that occurs without pain to the person) at some point in the past years. Most likely, this happened prior to one of his ER visits.

CAROTID INTIMA-MEDIA THICKNESS (CIMT)

This is a specialized ultrasound test that uses sound waves, not radiation, to measure the thickness of the internal lining of the carotid arteries. This test is a good indicator of your risk of a stroke or heart attack. The carotids branch out from the aorta, which is the major blood vessel that brings oxygenated blood from your heart to the rest of your body. The carotids are fed first, delivering oxygen to both sides of your brain. The walls of the carotids thicken due to inflammation, and though these arteries originate outside the heart, they're still a reflection of what might be going on inside—obstruction within the coronary arteries due to plaque, for instance. By restricting bloodflow to the brain, you have less oxygenated blood going to your head. When the coronary artery is obstructed by plaque, you may have a heart attack; alternatively, when the carotid arteries are blocked by plaque, you may have a stroke if a clot breaks out.

PULMONARY FUNCTION

These tests measure how much you exhale to figure out what the trouble could be, such as asthma, bronchitis, or emphysema. They are administered by having you breathe forcefully into a tube. You shouldn't eat a heavy meal before the test or smoke 4 to 6 hours prior. Your doctor will tell you whether or not to use inhalers prior to the test if you're already on them.

COMPUTED TOMOGRAPHY CALCIUM (CT-Ca)

These non-invasive tests look for calcium deposits in the coronary arteries that can narrow your arteries and increase your heart attack risk. The CT-Ca measures your past history of plaque and the calcium deposits within it. The result is a calcium score, which is the number of deposits, literally: Is it 10 or 550? If there are too many deposits, the overall coronary vessels may be obscured on the scan, making it difficult to get an accurate reading of soft plaque (which is telling with regard to how much the vessel is actually obstructed). The degree of plaque that's calcified, giving you your calcium score, is predictive of the amount of plaque in your body and your future risk of a heart attack in comparison to other men your age and demographic. Many doctors believe that calcified plaque, or stable plaque, will not cause a heart attack because it's hardened. Soft plaque is apparently worrisome, as it is evolving and mobile. A more invasive study, like a cardiac catheterization, may be recommended if your doctor feels it necessary to better determine your risk of a heart attack.

COMPUTED TOMOGRAPHY CORONARY ANGIOGRAM (CT-a)

This imaging test looks at the arteries that supply your heart muscle with blood to see if they've narrowed, causing chest pain or putting you at risk for a heart attack. Unlike a traditional coronary angiogram, CT angiograms don't use a catheter threaded through your blood vessels to your heart. Instead, a coronary CT angiogram relies on a powerful x-ray machine to produce 3D images of your heart and heart vessels. They don't require the recovery time needed with traditional angiograms and are a common option for people with a variety of heart conditions. A downside is that CT angiograms will expose you to a small amount of radiation—about what you get daily in a big city or on a cross-country flight. If you have known coronary artery disease, and may need intervention, a traditional coronary angiogram may be a better option that allows for angioplasty (balloon placement or stents to hold the vessel open). However, a CT-a is definitely the way to go if you're using it for screening purposes. With the results, you can best determine whether any of your risk factors (elevated cholesterol and/or sugar, low testosterone, positive family history, high blood pressure) is leading to plaque that is blocking ideal bloodflow through your coronary arteries.

You will receive instructions from your doctor on what to expect before going in for testing. This will include information on how soon you will need to cease eating and drinking before getting your CT angiogram, and what medications, like beta blockers, you may be given to improve the clarity of the scan by slowing your heart rate temporarily.

These heart scans may show that you have a higher risk of having a heart attack or other problems before you have any obvious symptoms of heart disease. While the American Heart Association and the American College of Cardiology do not advocate heart scans for individuals who don't have any symptoms of heart disease, sometimes there's no way to tell what's going on at a deeper level without these scans. You might have to explore this further with your doctor because it's not routine. Remember Tim Russert didn't have a CT-a of his heart, but he certainly had risk factors for cardiovascular disease like high cholesterol and obesity. Had he received a CT-a, he might not have died at 58. There was even a debate in the media after he died about why this test was not performed, as Tim had many known risk factors for a heart attack.

PULMONARY COMPUTED TOMOGRAPHY (PULMONARY CT)

Checking your lungs makes sense if you are a smoker, have been a smoker, or have been exposed to smoke from a partner or parents steadily over years. You might also elect this test if you have lived abroad with a chance of being exposed to TB or if lung cancer runs in your family. Bartenders have high risk of secondhand smoke exposure, though now that smoking laws have changed, this situation has improved. Still, 10 to 15 percent of people who die of lung cancer have never smoked. Exposure and genetics might be the cause.

An excellent benefit of this test is that lung cancer can be detected well before symptoms emerge. I also like this test because it's minimally invasive: It requires only an IV to inject the contrast dye that helps the doctor see if there's an unusual spot in the lungs. It is possible to get a pulmonary CT along with the coronary CT; given that the heart lies over the lungs, technically the radiologist can screen simultaneously. Speak to your doctor about going this route if you are at risk and focused on prevention.

LIPID METABOLISM

Testing the lipid subclasses (particle size and density), will be standard in the years to come. You might need further testing of these cholesterol particles even if your total and LDL test results were fine. Do you have heart disease in your family? Was your cholesterol in range? If you answered yes to both, here's a little more on why that might be.

One of the great mysteries of cardiology is the fact that 50 percent of people with coronary artery disease have blood cholesterol levels similar to those of people who do not develop the disease. One study of more than 17,000 people with low LDL (bad) cholesterol levels showed that a surprising number of them still developed heart disease. Inflammation, which is reflected in your cardiac-CRP and homocysteine scores, often plays a role in cardiovascular risk even if cholesterol is within range. Still, routine cholesterol tests are failing to identify the majority of people who are at risk for heart attacks. Figuring out the ratio between "good" and "bad" cholesterol is simply not enough to identify individuals at risk. To get some answers, I've begun to look deeper. Bad cholesterol is known as LDL; however, you can subdivide this measure further into small and large LDL particles. You want more of the bigger, buoyant LDL particles because they are larger and less likely to cause plaque buildup.

Insist upon a discussion of this more advanced blood work with your physician to maximize the prevention of coronary artery disease. The following comprehensive panel can detect inherited abnormalities that are beyond the reach of conventional HDL and LDL analysis. It can also indicate, at a genetic level, if the medications, supplements, and lifestyle choices you have made will actually work to reverse or prevent heart disease in your individual situation. This step takes priority, though it may not be necessary for everybody. Depending on the reason for getting these additional lipid tests, insurance would likely cover it.

LDL IIIA+B, LDL IVB—SMALL LDL PARTICLES

Small LDL particles come in two varieties: LDL IIIa+b and LDL IVb. Both are bad and result in faster accumulation of plaque. Medications along with a healthy lifestyle can help reduce this number. Ideally, you want to have a low LDL, which is mostly large LDL particles. For most folks, however, it's usually more of a mixed bag.

HDL2B—LARGE HDL PARTICLES

You already know that HDL is good cholesterol, and HDL2b measures the amount of larger HDL particles. The larger the HDL particles, the better. Your blood vessels are loosely woven. Large HDL particles block the spaces and prevent LDL from going inside and getting stuck, eventually leading to the arterial narrowing. While they aren't as protective as HDL2b, small HDL particles are rather neutral.

APOB—LDL PARTICLE NUMBER

ApoB is a component of LDL, in that however much ApoB you have is telling us how much LDL and VLDL (very low-density lipoprotein) you have. ApoB is a more precise biomarker than LDL, as LDL is calculated based on a formula and not measured directly.

LP(A) EXTENDED RANGE

Lp(a) is a component of LDL cholesterol, however, levels of Lp(a) are genetically predetermined. If Lp(a) is high, you likely will have a genetically higher risk of LDL cholesterol. Once you have this information, it's to your benefit. Statin therapy is generally recommended for this finding. You can take more preventive steps by adjusting your diet and exercise according to my recommendations. If Lp(a) is very elevated, then you have to work harder at keeping everything in check. This number will not change much throughout your lifetime—it's pretty set.

LP-PLA2—INFLAMMATION IN THE ARTERY

Lp-PLA2 is a very acute marker of inflammation. If I got a blood test back and the result was an Lp-PLA2 of 300 ng/mL, which is quite elevated, I would probably give that patient a call immediately. While inflammation within heart vessels is the likely trigger, other sources of inflammation in the body might also cause an elevated Lp-PLA2. Regardless, I would want to further evaluate possible reasons for the elevated level.

FIBRINOGEN—INFLAMMATION MARKER AND CLOTTING FACTOR

Fibrinogen is another inflammatory marker that indicates risk for heart disease.

NT-PROBNP—STRESS ON THE HEART

NT-proBNP is something that's followed very closely in people with heart failure, and it correlates with the amount of excess fluid in your body. If it's elevated, you probably already know that you have heart failure. Most people present with symptoms and don't necessarily need this test to tell them something is wrong; however, it offers confirmation.

THYROID FUNCTION

Your thyroid is typically examined during a physical exam, especially if you have symptoms indicative of low or high thyroid hormone secretion. If the thyroid is large or irregular on either side, further testing such as a thyroid ultrasound is recommended.

Lab test results may also be out of range for TSH, T3, T4, or any combination, which I typically will obtain at baseline analysis. I might recommend a medication to balance a thyroid that is underactive. Thyroid activity is complex, and the relationship between these three factors may be indicative of various etiologies.

I also might use iodine to assess iodine deficiency, especially if you have a higher TSH with low T3 or T4 indicating hypothyroidism. I can test for iodine inadequacy; however, it involves 2 days of urine testing, which is often not feasible. It is generally easier for individuals to try iodine supplementation. The iodine should help elevate T3 levels, allowing the thyroid hormones to optimize and TSH to drop.

I would also measure thyroid antibodies via further blood work to determine if you have an immune system abnormality like Hashimoto's disease, or thyroiditis. Various findings dictate different approaches; some involve monitoring, while others involve intervention with supplements or medication.

The thyroid ultrasound is a separate test used to detect Hashimoto's and Graves' disease. It may also be used to evaluate an abnormal thyroid on exam or nodules on your thyroid. If nodules are seen, you would want to undergo a stereotactic biopsy to determine if there are any abnormal cells in them. Should tests reveal further workup is indicated or medications fail to normalize thyroid function over a given amount of time, then the next step would be a referral to an endocrinologist by your doctor.

LIVER FUNCTION

In Chapter 3, we looked at how your body processes waste, specifically through the function of the liver. If the liver function tests came back with an abnormal reading, you may want to do further testing to see how much support the liver needs to do its job. Viral markers can detect the presence of hepatitis C and any prior exposure to other forms of hepatitis, like hepatitis A or B. An ultrasound of the liver can tell your doctor if there are fatty deposits, an indicator of more serious liver disease. If your doctor suspects cirrhosis—and you don't have to be an alcoholic to have this—or cancer, then you may need a biopsy.

ADVANCED IMAGING AND HIGHLY INDIVIDUALIZED BLOOD TESTS

IF YOUR COMPLETE BLOOD COUNT (CBC) ISN'T QUITE RIGHT . . .

Larry N. (Chapter 3) had a complete blood count that showed very elevated lymphocyte levels and low neutrophil levels, indicative of an immune system disorder. In his case, it led to a diagnosis of leukemia. At this point, as I did with Larry, I refer to a specialist, typically a hematologist who may run additional blood tests and initiate further workup.

IF YOUR PROSTATE IS ENLARGED, YOUR PROSTATE SCORE IS HIGH, OR YOU ARE AT RISK FOR PROSTATE CANCER...

If you've been to the doctor regularly, you've been monitoring your PSA for years. What's important to look at besides the total PSA number is the percentage of free PSA in your bloodstream. A higher percent free PSA has been associated with prostate cancer.

IF YOU HAVE ELEVATED HOMOCYSTEINE...

If an elevated homocysteine level is found on your initial lab tests, it would be important to measure your vitamin B_{12} and folate levels in your body. These are simple, follow-up lab tests that involve drawing blood as you did with your original evaluation. Vitamin B_{12} levels are typically 200 to 1,000 picograms per milliliter (pg/mL), and ideally, greater than 400 pg/mL. At levels lower than 400 pg/mL, there is a risk of cognitive decline and memory loss as you age.

As you progress with changes in your lifestyle, your homocysteine level may rise initially before it lowers. If you're being truly compliant—you're getting plenty of sleep, you've reduced your stress, you're working out four or five sessions a week, and your food intake is adjusted for optimal health—then this can actually be a good sign. It can mean that you're using up your vitamin B_{12} and folate more rapidly than before, and your body may not be able to keep up with the demand. You'll want to continue eating healthy and supplement with the FloQi supplements that have greens and fruit powders (see Chapter 8).

If your homocysteine does not respond to these changes, you will want to consider a blood test to determine if you have an aberrant gene, termed MTHFR. If you have this gene, you won't be able to metabolize enough folate from food or oral supplements for your cellular function. Folks with this finding, which is relatively common, have a higher risk of clots associated with thromboembolic events (like deep vein thrombosis, also called DVT, with risk of a pulmonary embolus) and twice the risk of a heart attack. Air travel can predispose to clot formation. If you have this gene, talk to your doctor about B_{12} injections as well as supplementation with other B-complex vitamins, especially folate.

ADVANCED GENETIC TESTS

Men, less commonly than women, will sometimes mention that they are "sensitive" to certain medications. Despite the fact that it is well known that people react differently to the same medication and dosage, up until recently, there has been little variation with regard to prescription guidelines. Now you can do better. There are ways to determine how you might handle certain medications, as well as over-the-counter pills such as aspirin. These tests detect the proper dosage and the risk versus benefit ratio for you. Several institutions, and individual physicians, have been utilizing genetic testing over the past decade to help manage patients with various conditions, ranging from medications for blood thinner (warfarin, or Coumadin) to depression (SSRIs). Certain tests will also tell you if you are at risk for a disease that other lab data may miss.

The following genetic factors, measured by Berkeley HeartLab, will aid in decision making regarding certain medications and will help give you an even more complete picture of your overall health.

9P21 GENOTYPE TEST

Maybe you're like Wayne Hickory, and you have a SNP on the 9p21 allele. This genetic mutation increases your risk for cardiovascular disease; however, you can mitigate this by eating a diet that is rich in raw fruits and vegetables.

APOE GENOTYPE TEST

ApoE tells you your risk for heart disease and potentially Alzheimer's as well. In Chapter 12, you'll see that Wade B. (from Chapter 6) decided to undergo this testing. He was very nervous about getting his results, because he was afraid they might show he was at risk for developing early-onset Alzheimer's.

KIF6 GENOTYPE TEST

If you have a mutation on the KIF6 gene, you're likely to have a better response to the statins, which are medications that doctors often prescribe if you have high cholesterol. This mutation, however, may also indicate you're at a higher risk for heart disease.

LPA-ASPIRIN GENOTYPE TEST

When I discussed aspirin in Chapter 8, I mentioned that there was a genetic test that would help determine whether or not you should take aspirin. People who are LPA-aspirin carriers are at a greater risk for heart disease, and aspirin may help lower that risk. If you don't test positive for this gene, then taking aspirin might pose a greater risk of bleeding, and that risk may outweigh any potential benefits like heart attack and stroke prevention. Nevertheless, many men might benefit from a daily low dose (81 mg) aspirin, an ideal example of the judgment that would be necessary to assess all the factors that would lead to cardiovascular diseases, such as heart attack or stroke.

LPA-INTRON 25 GENOTYPE TEST

LPA-Intron tells you if you have a higher genetic predisposition to have elevated cholesterol. You may have to work harder than the average person to keep your cholesterol low. Your genes are against you, though they can be altered via epigenetics! Stay tuned.

SLCO1B1 GENOTYPE TEST

If you carry SLCO1B1, you may have increased muscle aches (myalgias and myopathies) if you take statins. In my patients who have this mutation, I often prescribe CoQ10, which helps to mitigate these side effects.

4Q25-AF RISK GENOTYPE

If you carry this gene, you're at an increased risk for atrial fibrillation, which is a cardiac arrhythmia. This is usually detected on EKG, or testing after a patient complains of feeling like his heart is skipping beats or its rhythm is irregular in some way. Some men have few or no symptoms at all, while others may be extremely symptomatic, with shortness of breath and weakness, necessitating a visit to the ER when atrial fibrillation presents suddenly.

When you take your tests, don't just file the results in a drawer. They are crucial information for charting your progress and improving your personal health metrics. If your stats are headed in a good direction, then you're moving toward your sweet spot for optimizing your health span and you are feeling better overall, too. But if your stats aren't showing improvement, or if they're going the wrong way, then use the information to adjust and individualize your program, be it sleep, food, exercise, supplements, or medications. In the next chapter, I'm going to show you how to put everything together to move you into your sweet spot. I will revisit some of the men from Chapters 3 and 4, and you will be able to see the progress they made after one year. Typically, men perceive an improved sense of well-being and sexual function within weeks, with clothes that fit differently, belts pulled tighter within a couple of months. Lab data confirms metabolic improvement in carb and lipid profiles as well as hormonal (testosterone, DHEA) optimization. Lean muscle and loss of fat follows at 10 to 12 weeks and is documented on a body comp test, along with measurable changes in VO_2 assessments at a follow-up visit. As these concrete biomarkers demonstrate palpable advances, my team and I rejoice along with our patient. It is an amazing feeling of accomplishment; then we set new objectives together to move to the next stage.

CHAPTER 11

ACHIEVING YOUR SWEET SPOT
These patients did, and you can, too

If you were to ask a successful person what's his goal, it's always to try and be better. It's not necessarily to try and make more money. If you have enough money, you don't have to define your-self by making money. It's to be better. Be better at the things that you do. Be better at how you treat people. And you don't lose your patience because you're able to deal with stress better. You just become better. Better at everything.

Being able to feel younger, I'm better. I'm not stressing over the aches and pains, the throwing my back out, the hurting myself, the stuff that I watch happen every day because people just don't take care of themselves.

If you think about it, this is the commitment: Can you take five pills a day? How long does it take to take five pills a day? Thirty seconds. If you need to take a shot [of hCG], and learn how

to do it yourself, how long does that take? Five minutes. Now
we're at 5 ½ minutes. Now work out for a total of 3 hours a week.
For slightly over 3 hours a week, you can have this. You can be
better. Three hours a week. That's your whole commitment.

—JOE NICOLLA, age 55, real estate company owner

B y this point, you realize that you're an individual, with a unique
history, a unique makeup that's different from your friends' and
maybe even from your brother's. There's no such thing as normal, and figuring out your own metabolic and hormonal blue-
print requires you to factor in all of your personal health metrics,
including medical history, lifestyle, family history, and lab results. My
hope is that you've invested some time digging into your history, as I
showed you in Chapter 2, and that you now have a clearer picture of
who you are today. You also may have gotten blood work done and now
have your baseline stats.

Once you understand your unique profile, you can begin to implement appropriate changes laid out for you in Chapters 5 through 7.
Depending on how you've been living, that might mean getting more
sleep and working out more; or eating breakfast; or keeping to a regular
schedule of meals and snacks; or engaging in stress reduction. Even if
you're doing a lot right, there's always going to be room to do more to
prevent the downward slide that comes with aging. My hope is that
Chapters 8 and 9 indicated a direction you might need to take with
regard to supplements and hormone treatment. A conversation with a
trusted health care clinician will help you identify what combination is
best for you to achieve optimal results. By this point, your doctor may also
want to recommend the advanced diagnostics described in Chapter 10.
For example, if you had a parent who died of a heart attack at a young
age, getting advanced tests like a CT-a with calcium score or CIMT
could prove lifesaving.

Having gotten this far, you are definitely in the game of retrieving
your health and optimizing your health span. This chapter will help you
hit that sweet spot. Once you get there, you'll be able to make the most

of my recommendations and advice and really turn things around. Remember Kirk Hansen from the Introduction? Thanks to the new diet, medications, and other recommendations I made, Kirk's body was primed to change for the better. But he let his workouts slide. He just needed to put in the work.

I can help you achieve your sweet spot, creating a process for you that will lead to capturing the energy and vitality that may now seem unattainable. This path will vary for each man; some of you may have to do more to reach it, and others will get by with less. Your makeup will dictate distinctive interventions and lead you to make different choices. These choices will differ from your best buddy's, even if he's your identical twin. Expect to be unique.

WHERE ARE YOU IN THE SCHEME OF THINGS?

It is important to understand where you are on the spectrum of health within each of these areas: sleep, stress, sex, food, and fitness. Making lifestyle changes is within your immediate control. If you can keep track of your lab results and your progress in each of these areas, you can judge where you are by the most important benchmark: how you measure up to yourself. That's what matters.

Take a look at how I've laid out the following five elements of good health: sleep, stress, sex, food, and fitness. Decide where you fall right now according to the descriptions of the grades listed below them. These are sliding scales; you can go up and down and be somewhere in between based on your lifestyle choices.

SLEEP

BLOODSHOT: Your sleep hygiene is terrible. You stay up far too late, you leave the TV on, you're texting throughout the night, you can't breathe when you do fall asleep. Even your pillow thinks you're pathetic.

SLEEPY DWARF: You're chronically tired. Maybe you're an insomniac, or perhaps you have sleep apnea. You're becoming more aware of your sleepiness and your need for more sleep.

ALMOST ENOUGH: You're like pretty much anybody you know—you sleep enough, but you wish you got more of it. Weekends are when you make up for lost time, but that's after you return at 3:00 a.m. from a night out on the town.

7- TO 8-HOUR SEMIPRO: You know that sleep is critical, and you make it a priority. You have a bedtime, and you tend to stick to it.

LIKE A BABY: Children get the best sleep out of any of us—it's consolidated, and they get a good amount of stage 3 and 4, the deep stuff. They also typically get 8 hours, if not much more. The closer we can get back to that sleep pattern, the better. If you're almost there, you're in good shape.

STRESS

FRAZZLED AND NUMB: Everything feels like it's just too much. You should care, but you're so overwhelmed you can't engage with anything. It's tough to get up off the couch.

MULTITASKING FIEND: Your cortisol is out of control. You're trying to run in 50 different directions with work obligations and carpooling and that yard work that keeps piling up. You're anxious and depressed, and the way you know this is that you overreact to pretty much everything.

MODERN CITIZEN: You manage to keep it together—barely—but you've got an electronic device on every surface at home and the office. Between your smartphone, tablet, desktop, and laptop, you're running on all platforms 24/7. Just because you're like most of the people you see, doesn't mean it's healthy.

SMOOTH AND EASY: You've got your priorities and you stick to them—you plan ahead and stay organized. There's bound to be something upsetting here and there, but you know how to take a deep breath and keep moving. You feel unruffled most of the time.

MEDITATION MASTER: The yogis are asking you for advice.

SEX

SOLO ARTIST: Masturbation is the only action you get, and it's not very satisfying.

TAKE THE MONEY AND RUN: The act is either infrequent, or your performance is lacking. Sometimes it's both.

DINNER AND A MOVIE AND...: Special occasions shouldn't be the only time you get intimate. Lately, you've decided every other Friday is date night. It's not ideal, but it's still better than what's going on for some of your friends.

COMMITTED: You're having sex twice per week, and getting some on the weekends, sometimes multiple times per day.

YOU WEAR A PERPETUAL SMILE: You're having great, satisfying sex as often as you like.

FOOD

MCDONALD'S VIP: Fast food, sweets, and soda are your staples. You often go long stretches without eating only to gorge when famished.

MICROWAVE MACHINE: Anything that's prepackaged or processed is your go-to sustenance: TV dinners, toaster pastries, canned pastas, anything that's quick and easy to heat and eat (and loaded with chemical preservatives).

GRANOLA GUY: You've got the basics of nutrition down. You're eating breakfast, getting enough protein, and staying hydrated. Meal timing is pretty good, but sometimes erratic.

THE GRASSHOPPER: You are eating more manageable meals throughout the day. You may need more protein to put on lean muscle or rev up nutrient intake as your body burns hotter; more energy being expended uses up B vitamins.

MASTER CHEF: You select and prepare the foods that are good for you and you eat throughout the day with remarkable regularity. You're prepared with snacks and healthy alternatives at parties and during travel.

FITNESS

CHANNEL SURFER: Walking to the beer cooler is your only cardiovascular training. Clicking the remote is your resistance training.

THE GUY FRIDAY: You put in little time at the gym during slow days at work, maybe a light jog or weights on the weekends.

BALANCING ACT: You've got some structured program, though one type of exercise may predominate. For instance, perhaps you prefer cardio over resistance training; you're a runner who just won't lift weights.

WORKMAN ATHLETE: It's in hand: structured program, regular workouts, balanced resistance, cardio, flexibility.

COMPETITOR/PRO: Well-planned regular workouts are designed to prepare your body for a specific event or events.

IN THE FOOTSTEPS OF OTHERS

As you've read the stories of the men in the book, perhaps you identified with one person or saw yourself as an amalgam of several patients—Cedric, Noah, and Stanley, let's say. The stories are intended to illuminate your own and inspire action, not to serve as stereotypes defining you by one trait or another. Nor are they there for you to compare yourself negatively. My hope is that they show you the possibilities and allow you to cherry-pick the details that help you understand how to increase your own health span.

Here's follow-up on several of the men you've been reading about. You can see what they did, where they needed help, and how they implemented change in their first year. While I may highlight one particular area of their lives, please do understand that these men, just like you, are not one-dimensional, nor did they have a single area in which they needed support. Many aspects of their entire being had to be taken into account.

By using their stories as examples, my goal is to help you to understand the diagnoses you may receive reflect your lifestyle choices and family history and are supported by lab data. A seemingly sudden gout attack has been brewing since you started drinking with clients three times a week 5 years ago. You find out your mother had gouty arthritis, too. By showing you what happened with each of these men, you might better understand how you can turn around your health.

TURNING AROUND RISK FACTORS FOR HEART DISEASE: CHOLESTEROL AND TRIGLYCERIDES

ETHAN H. was the gentleman who was so uncomfortable with his body shape that he feared physical intimacy. In Chapter 4, I introduced Ethan as someone who had hypothyroidism that had gone undiagnosed for years—low free T3 and T4, yet a TSH that was within range. He's also a good example of someone whose cardiovascular risk was mounting.

Problems

- Borderline high cholesterol

- Elevated homocysteine and cardiac-CRP

- Borderline prediabetes

- Hypothyroidism

- Low T

Corrections

- His overall cholesterol had been high at 209 mg/dL and his LDL (bad cholesterol) was elevated at 119 mg/dL. The good news was that his triglycerides and HDL (good cholesterol) were fine. Within 6 months, his total cholesterol was 189 mg/dL, while his LDL was still over 100 mg/dL.

- Because his LDL hadn't changed significantly and there were additional signs of inflammation, like an elevated homocysteine and cardiac-CRP, I decided to put him on a low dose of Crestor. This is a statin designed to lower cholesterol and also has been shown to reduce inflammation.

- He added adequate protein to his meals, regulated his food intake, and cut back on the wine at dinner as well as the desserts. His prediabetic status improved within 3 months.

- I started thyroid hormone to increase his T3 levels and improve his metabolism.

- I immediately started him on omegas-3s and fruit and vegetable powders to help improve his nutrient levels.

- I added twice-weekly self-injections of hCG to boost testosterone and improve his ability to put on muscle.

Improvements

Ethan was able to improve his cholesterol levels and his weight. He responded to the statin Crestor remarkably well, his LDL dropping to 61 mg/dL and total cholesterol falling to 132 mg/dL. His cardiac-CRP was under 1 (it was 0.6, which is great), thereby reducing his risk for cardiovascular disease. Due to his diet and exercise, his triglycerides halved for the first time.

A note on statins: The Jupiter study, the clinical trial I mentioned in Chapter 3, showed that rosuvastatin (Crestor) actually helped to lower cardiac-CRP in patients who had low-to-normal cholesterol levels but elevated c-CRPs, indicating inflammation. While the study was intended to last 5 years, it was halted before the 2-year mark because the benefit of statins was shown to be so significant. They couldn't justify giving placebos to half of the study's participants. On average, the drug reduced LDL levels by 50 percent and c-CRP by 37 percent. Additionally, there was a 60 percent decrease in the number of cardiac events—heart attack and sudden death—as well as a 70 percent decrease in stroke. A follow-up analysis showed that statins did increase the incidence of diabetes; however, the prevention of cardiovascular disease was determined to outweigh this risk.

Once I got Ethan moving, he progressed at the gym fairly rapidly, encouraged by the results he was seeing physically. He was religious about his nutrition, taking my suggestions and making adjustments when needed. His body composition changed significantly, a direct result of his new outlook on diet and exercise. Ethan started with an overall body fat of 35.5 percent and 27.7 percent in his trunk, both values higher than what I would like to see. Within a year, he had brought those numbers down to 22.2 percent and 21.8 percent, respectively. In total, he lost 36 pounds of fat and gained 5 pounds of muscle. After beginning hCG treatment, he was better able to put on lean muscle as his testosterone levels improved.

Challenges and Next Steps

Unfortunately, Ethan's stress increased, too, because work was fairly demanding. The difference was he felt like he could handle it. The bigger issue was helping Ethan to keep his motivation so that he would continue making gains following his initial success on the program. The good news was that he was becoming comfortable in his own skin.

DAVE R. had a strong family history of cardiovascular disease (his father had recently suffered a stroke) and high cholesterol. Look into your own medical history or ask a few of your buddies, and you'll find this combination is fairly common and also dangerous. Not only did Dave have a family history, his own tests indicated high cardiovascular risk. If you recall from Chapter 3, his triglycerides were so high that his LDL couldn't be calculated. At the same time, however, Dave had an almost insatiable desire to be active. As he searched for a new sport, I helped get his heart health in order.

Problems

- Triglyceride levels so high that his LDL (bad cholesterol) couldn't be calculated on the first go-around
- High blood pressure
- Low testosterone
- Poor sugar values—risk of gout indicated with elevated uric acid in lab data

Corrections

I immediately sent Dave in for advanced particle testing at Berkeley HeartLab (Chapter 10). This testing would give me a better appreciation for the types of particles that were making up Dave's LDL and HDL. To review, in general the large, fluffier particles are good; the small, sticky particles are bad because they tend to glom together and cause blockage and consequently inflammation. I also suggested he get a CT-a, CT-Ca, and CIMT to look for plaque and blockages in his cardiac vessels. It was imperative to get Dave's cholesterol under control even before his lab data came back.

I started Dave on Crestor and also once-daily baby aspirin after genetic testing determined the benefits of using each outweighed the risk. I supplemented these medications with L-arginine and L-citrulline to help improve vascular flow.

I also included:

- CoQ10, omegas, juice powders, alpha-lipoic acid, selenium, and CLA

- hCG initially and later injectable testosterone once he hit andropause

All this was a lot to throw at Dave, especially because he had never taken any medications. He was an athlete who always thought his stamina would keep illness at bay. In addition to monitoring the progress he made with his coach, I also encouraged him to eat more regularly throughout the day and cut back on foods with a high purine content—red wine, aged cheese, shellfish, sweets, spinach—to avoid attacks of gout (see Chapter 7).

Improvements

Within 3 months, Dave's triglycerides halved to 180 mg/dL. His total cholesterol was 150 mg/dL and his LDL was 70 mg/dL. His HDL remained low at 35 mg/dL. All in all, though, it was a terrific improvement, and it happened in less than 6 months. Dave found it difficult to get down the timing of his meals. As a result, his diabetes didn't improve as much as I had hoped. His hemoglobin A1c actually increased over time. On a positive note, Dave's risk of gout did improve, he cut back on purine-rich food and his uric acid level fell. Sleep had also surfaced as an issue during our follow-up appointments, so I wanted Dave to try SleepImage at home.

Challenges and Next Steps

Dave needs to improve his sleep and keep his diabetes risk in check, yet I have no doubt he'll do it. Dave is one of those guys who wants everything sooner, better, faster. He's doing great on the program, and his hard work is paying off.

The Takeaways

If your doctor tells you your cholesterol is high, that doesn't mean much unless you know more about your good and bad cholesterol, HDL and LDL (see Chapter 3). Ethan and Dave's total cholesterol levels were high; they also had low levels of good cholesterol and high levels of bad cholesterol. Additionally, their lipid profiles at the particle level were not good. Many people who have heart attacks are found to have unfavorable particles in spades. If your cholesterol levels are high, especially LDL, your doctor may have already started you on Lipitor. I prefer Crestor because it's been shown to raise HDL in addition to reducing LDL, as well as lowering c-CRP. Some supplements you may want to take include omega-3 fish oil (see Chapter 8), and if you prefer not to take a prescription statin, red yeast rice would be an option. It's imperative to start looking below the surface and exploring beyond total cholesterol levels.

TURNING AROUND OTHER RISK FACTORS FOR HEART DISEASE: INFLAMMATORY MARKERS

GREG M. had recently opened his own restaurant and was the primary caretaker for two young girls. Stress was a constant in his life, and his tests showed arterial inflammation. I needed to find out what was causing it and determine the severity of his risk for heart disease.

Problems

- Inflammatory markers homocysteine and cardiac-CRP were high at 8.2 pmol/L and 4.3 mg/L, respectively

- Gout attack—if you recall, he ate well, yet spinach omelettes were his go-to breakfast

- Low testosterone

Corrections

- Given his elevated inflammatory markers, I sent Greg in for advanced testing, which included Berkeley HeartLab's particle testing and a

CIMT, which would measure the medial thickness of his carotid arteries. If the walls of the arteries get thicker, they narrow the internal passage and that slows bloodflow; I aim for the walls to be narrow and the passage to be wide. Both tests came back abnormal, indicating that Greg's arterial walls were too thick. His Berkley HeartLab testing showed that he had unfavorable sticky, small LDL particles, contributing to his bad cholesterol.

- I started Greg on Crestor and aspirin, a combination that has been shown to be effective in reducing cardiac-CRP.

- Omegas, juice powder, D_3, melatonin

- Started on hCG

Improvements

At one year, Greg had lowered his cardiac-CRP to 0.8 mg/L. In tandem with his lifestyle changes, I supplemented Greg's diet with omegas, juice powder, vitamin D_3, melatonin, and FloQi Prime Power as well as Prime Alpha MicroTabs.

Early on during treatment, Greg had a gout attack in his left big toe, as his uric acid was 8.7 mg/dL (up from 7.1 mg/dL). In addition to advising him to alter his diet, I also started Greg on metformin. In subsequent lab data, I found Greg had borderline elevated hemoglobin A1c as well as fasting glucose and insulin. Metformin would address his borderline diabetes, which may have contributed to his cardiovascular risk. I switched Greg from hCG to testosterone, as he showed less responsiveness to the hCG, meaning that his testes weren't responding to the signals to produce testosterone. His LH was high, and yet his testes seemed to be ignoring this wake-up call from his brain to produce testosterone, and his testosterone levels remained low. High LH levels often signify andropause, so I started him on injectable depo-testosterone. That helped, yet it also increased his estradiol, which is produced from testosterone in fat. I prescribed anastrozole (Arimidex) to block the conversion of testosterone to estradiol and help reduce circulating estrogen. I added DHEA supplement to help bring testosterone levels up as well. (DHEA, if you recall, is a building block to testosterone.)

Challenges and Next Steps

Unfortunately, things at home were getting worse as his daughters began to hit puberty and act out. His father, a huge help to Greg at the restaurant, also passed away. Greg was meditating and using yoga to control his stress and continued to run and lift weights when he could find a spare moment.

The Takeaways

In general, if your labs reveal a cardiac-CRP that's above 5 mg/L, this is usually indicative of some kind of infection, injury, or inflammation. Recall from Chapter 3 that a very high cardiac-CRP could reflect an acute problem, like a broken arm or sinusitis, or it could be indicative of a more chronic condition like arthritis. When it's between 1 and 5 mg/L, then it's usually related to underlying cardiovascular disease. You may have inflammation in the walls of your arteries. The first step is to figure out the reason behind an elevated c-CRP. A CIMT is a good test to assess the degree of inflammation inside the lining of the carotid arteries. The next step would be getting a CT-Ca and CT-a to determine the amount of plaque and blockage in the coronary arteries (see Chapter 10). Aspirin would be your first line of defense for an elevated c-CRP. You might consider adding food high in omegas (see Chapter 7) and going heavier on the fruits and vegetables. Omega-3 supplements would also be useful.

BALANCING HORMONES, LIFE IMPROVEMENT

NOAH N. Turning 60 made Noah decide to take a long, hard look at his health and make some significant changes. He had high levels of the stress hormone cortisol and low testosterone. Stress, though difficult to quantify at times, has a huge impact on a person's ability to function, get enough rest, and stay in shape. For several years, the weight around Noah's middle had been inching up. The demands of working on an action film—the early morning calls, the extra takes, the adjustment to life working on set in a foreign country instead of LA—were making his anxiety worse. He was neither sleeping nor eating right. His labs showed that while his fasting sugar and insulin were in the reference range, his hemoglobin A1c was 5.9 percent, indicating that he was prediabetic.

Problems:

- Very high cortisol at 24 mcg/dL, helping to explain why his abs were looking more like a belly

- Low total and free testosterone levels—309 ng/dL and 49 pg/mL, respectively

- Low DHEA, which probably contributed to his low T

- Low IGF-1, likely connected in part to his lack of good quality sleep

- Low Vitamin D

- Reoccurring gastric ulcers, a problem that ran in his family

Corrections

I wanted to help Noah lower his stress levels and, by association, his cortisol. He had to put in the energy to improve his sleep and take more time to unwind and relax. He began practicing yoga regularly, and I suggested he try GABA wafers, which act on the brain to improve concentration. (GABA is an amino acid in the brain that acts as the chief inhibitory neurotransmitter, promoting a calmer mood. It also is responsible for maintaining muscle tone.) To reduce his hemoglobin A1c, he was eating smaller meals more consistently throughout the day, also ramping up his protein consumption.

I also prescribed Metformin to manage his poor carbohydrate metabolism. (I later found out the Noah couldn't tolerate it, after he experienced several bouts of diarrhea.)

Improvements

Within 6 months, Noah's cortisol had dropped to 14 mcg/dL, and at a year, it was at 7 mcg/dL—a marked improvement from 24 mcg/dL.

Within 1 year, Noah's free testosterone was at optimal levels, and his IGF-1 also rebounded. As his free testosterone went up, however, DHT rose with it. I put Noah on saw palmetto (Chapter 8), which lowers DHT, with good results. In addition to prescribing testosterone injections, I supplemented with DHEA and vitamin D. I added aspirin to decrease risk of cardiovascular disease as well as to offset some of the damage that smoking did to his body. On a positive note, Noah had significant fat loss, gained lean muscle, and his waist size went back to where he was in college. He did end up with a new wardrobe at the end of the year.

Challenges and Next Steps

Noah never managed to quit smoking. Still hasn't. This contributes to multiple risks, including cancers (throat, lung, bladder, esophageal, and others), cardiovascular disorders, and inflammatory conditions. He says it helps ease his anxiety, yet he knows it's a crutch he's relied on for too long.

TONY N. was in free fall. As I was getting ready to call to warn him about his risks based on his initial lab data, he had a stroke.

Problems

His lab results showed that he had elevated total cholesterol and LDL, and a 2-hour glucose tolerance test confirmed that he also had borderline diabetes. My main concern was the numbers in his hormone panel, however. Nothing looked very good.

- Low total and free testosterone—296 ng/dL and 78 pg/mL, respectively

- His DHEA was low at 137 ng/dL, and his cortisol was high at 19 mcg/dL, making it difficult for him to lose weight around the middle despite going on extreme diets and working out regularly.

- His low vitamin D likely may be one of several factor that contributed to his stroke and cardiovascular disease.

- Of significance, Tony's PSA was high at 4.5 ng/mL. In Chapter 4, I detailed the main reasons why PSA may be elevated: (1) acute prostatitis; (2) an enlarged prostate, known as benign prostatic hyperplasia (BPH); (3) prostate cancer.

Corrections

Because Tony's PSA was high, I referred him to a urologist. The urologist biopsied Tony's prostate and found he had option 2: BPH. We started him on hCG to optimize his testosterone. Additionally, I put him on Avodart, a medication that's used to treat BPH. Vitamin D_2, Cialis, B_{12} injections, Glucophage for his diabetes, CoQ10, DHEA, melatonin, L-arginine and L-ornithine, alpha-lipoic acid, omega-3, and juice powders in FloQi Prime Power were among his other medications and supplements.

Improvements

His rigorous adherence to my recommendations, including the start of Crestor, also helped him to turn around his cholesterol numbers—his total cholesterol, triglycerides, and LDL all decreased by 50 percent. His HDL increased, too.

Challenges and Next Steps

For someone that is physically active, the hard transition is going from doing something to doing nothing. Tony was a gym rat, and he found it challenging to slow down after his stroke. In fact, I had to suggest that he start physical therapy, and the rehabilitation process took months. After a stroke, you reduce the free range of motion to whatever area was injured. Depending on the extent of the damage, this impairment may last a long time or be permanent. Scheduling appointments with a physical therapist is critical. What you may not realize is the physical therapy is a structured rehabilitation workout, and it's not necessarily easy.

Once Tony was ready to go back to the gym, I steered him in a better direction. Before his stroke, he was training incorrectly. This is common, especially with resistance training. I started him on a cycle ergometer due to the previous lack of balance in his exercise regimen (too much lifting, not enough cardio), and soon thereafter I set him up with a personal trainer.

Given his recent stroke, I took an approach that was as aggressive in discovery as possible. I wanted to ensure such an event wouldn't happen again. The results from Berkeley HeartLab showed that he was heterozygous for the 9p21 gene, increasing his risk for cardiovascular disease. A SNP in his SLCO1B1 gene showed him to have a higher risk for myopathy, which was important to know given he was on statins. Based upon these results, I wanted to get him started on baby aspirin once daily and also scheduled additional testing, including a CT-a, CT-Ca, and CIMT.

The Takeaways

Almost all the men that I see start out by having testosterone levels that are less than optimal. Noah and Tony were no exceptions, and their hormone panels revealed other troubling finds. Noah had extremely high cortisol, and several values in Tony's hormone panel were out of range, namely vitamin D and PSA. With this knowledge, however, I was able to craft personalized medical interventions and promote positive lifestyle changes that reversed their risk of burnout and cardiovascular disease. Their health spans are predicted to increase based on their test scores. Most importantly, both report a significant improvement in their quality of life.

Remember, hormones underpin systemic function. You should get your levels tested as soon as possible so that you can establish a baseline and begin making changes. More exercise and better sleep may boost your growth hormone level. Practicing regular stress relief may help improve your cortisol. DHEA supplementation can help raise testosterone levels, as DHEA is a precursor to T.

BOOSTING YOUR ABILITY TO TURN FOOD INTO FUEL: CARBOHYDRATE METABOLISM

LIVINGSTON MILLER is the personal trainer with a model's body who appeared in an ad for the New York City gym where he worked. If you recall, however, Livingston collapsed during a golf game and had to be rushed to the hospital.

Problems

- Borderline diabetic. His hemoglobin A1c wasn't terrible—5.9 percent—but it was already affecting his heart.

- Silent heart attack, which led to a diagnosis of anterior wall hypokinesis (poor heart muscle motion)

- Frequent urination

- Low testosterone and DHEA

Corrections

To help Livingston manage his prediabetic condition, I started him on metformin. He continued to complain to me that his belly felt distended no matter what he did. I told him it was likely because he worked out all the time, he ate too many carbs, was a wine lover, and wasn't getting enough protein. So he switched up his diet to include more lean meats and reduced his alcohol consumption. Putting on muscle was *not* something that Livingston needed, so as you read in Chapter 7, I had him incorporate more aerobic exercise into his routine to help his heart.

Given his low testosterone levels. I also started him on testosterone, which improved his performance all around. Because his DHEA was below range, I started him on a DHEA supplement, which helped to increase the levels circulating in his body, thereby promoting testosterone production.

Improvements

- He had a very nice response to the metformin: his hemoglobin A1c dropped to 5.6 percent, his fasting glucose went from 92 to 80 mg/dL, and his fasting insulin went from 5 to 2 μIU/mL.

- Improvements in diet and workout led to a 20-pound weight loss, mostly evident around his trunk. His body composition scan showed this change. Previously, he was doing weights without much cardiovascular exercise except for the limited walking on his golf games Saturday and Sunday. Once he ramped up his aerobic activity, his weight dropped further, and his personal metrics improved.

Challenges and Next Steps

Livingston still enjoyed a glass of red wine several times a week and had difficulty cutting back. If he adjusted his lifestyle, I hoped to see an even greater reduction in his hemoglobin A1c.

STANLEY W. is the college professor who started to take stock of his current health when he began training with our exercise physiologist. He had a doctor who said his hemoglobin A1c of 7.7 percent was nothing to worry about, when the data are clear that a value of 6.0 percent is the cutoff for diabetes.

Problems

He was on an inadequate amount of metformin, as confirmed by a 2-hour glucose tolerance test, which showed that his carbohydrate metabolism was still abnormal. His numbers were way too high. His indulgent lifestyle filled with generous amounts of rich, carb-heavy foods, and alcohol was also hindering his progress. He also had low testosterone; he was experiencing problems in sexual function and suffered from depression.

Corrections

- Helped him get better results at the gym by having our exercise physiologist design a program that was tailored to his metabolic profile
- Upped his dose of metformin
- Started him on Victoza, a glucagon-like peptide that helps to make him feel full and balances his insulin. By keeping blood sugar in check, this once-a-day injection helps Stan keep his cravings under control.
- Started testosterone

Improvements

- Upping the dose of metformin helped lower Stan's fasting glucose to 90 mg/dL, his fasting insulin to 5 μIU/mL, and his hemoglobin A1c to 6.1 percent—and this was all in 6 months. Combined with his workouts at the gym, the medication helped Stan lose weight. Finally, his resistance training was giving him the lean muscle he wanted after I started on him testosterone, and, as a result, he was able to ramp up his aerobic exercise.

Challenges and Next Steps

Stan's lifestyle prevents him from getting all the results he desires. He hasn't cut back on his alcohol consumption, thereby limiting his future progress. He has to watch out as wine has a high sugar content. If he's going to drink, it's best if he pairs it with meals or a protein-rich snack like nuts to reduce sugar and insulin spikes. Lately, he has been making a concerted effort to cut back, and it's working.

The Takeaways

If you find on your lab tests that your numbers are close to Livingston's and Stan's, you may consider doing a 2-hour glucose tolerance test (see Chapter 10 to further evaluate your sugar metabolism). You also may want to ask your doctor about starting on metformin, then adding Byetta, Victoza, Symlin, or some combination thereof to manage your diabetes. My main choice of medication for prediabetics and those who already have type 2 diabetes is metformin because it's administered orally, is generally well-tolerated, and also has been shown to bring down cholesterol and triglycerides. Weight loss is often a secondary benefit to taking metformin. Recent data suggests it also decreases the production of inflammatory markers from aging cells.

Some useful supplements may be cinnamon and selenium; L-arginine can also help with the underlying vascular inflammation (see Chapter 8). And of course, cut back on the gratuitous carbs, balance carbs with protein, and keep moving. If you're not exercising regularly, you may want to begin with low intensity cardiovascular training. Remember, too, everyone's body reacts differently, and that's true even if you have an identical diagnosis, like diabetes. In these examples, Livingston was pre-diabetic and he was passing out from blood sugar crashes. Stan's numbers were much worse, but he didn't report the same symptoms.

GETTING YOUR COMPLETE BLOOD COUNT NUMBERS TO ADD UP

CEDRIC W. came in with anemia, which is unusual in a man. Without an obvious reason for blood loss, like recent surgery, you should have a colonoscopy done to make sure you're not bleeding internally, which may indicate cancer. The GI doctor who ran the colonoscopy on Cedric found nothing significant, so I determined that he either wasn't getting enough iron or his body wasn't able to absorb it properly or adequately.

Problems

- Severely low iron and ferritin levels
- Hematocrit and hemoglobin were under threshold.
- B_{12} and folate deficiency, indicating his body wasn't absorbing these minerals either
- I did an additional blood test, and the shape and color of his blood cells also pointed to a severe iron deficiency.
- Elevated homocysteine and cardiac-CRP
- Advanced genetic testing (see Chapter 10) was recommended due the elevated homocysteine. The test revealed that he carried the MTHFR gene. Men who have this variation are at greater cardiovascular risk and should be taking B supplements to counteract the increased odds for developing blood clots (deep vein thrombosis) and experiencing heart attacks.

Corrections

- I started supplementing with iron, B_{12}, and folate and also had him eat more vegetables and fruit to improve his homocysteine.

ACHIEVING YOUR SWEET SPOT

- The supplements I started included red yeast rice (to help lower his cholesterol), DHEA, and glucosamine/chondroitin/MSM (to help with joint function).

- I prescribed Ambien to help him get more regular sleep, especially after so many flights spanning disparate time zones. I eventually sent him home with our SleepImage testing (see Chapter 5), which revealed that he had interrupted sleep and snoring. An overnight study at a sleep lab confirmed moderate sleep apnea.

Improvements

- One year later, his iron and ferritin levels showed marked improvements—139 mcg/dL and 69 ng/mL, respectively. His hemoglobin was 16.6 and his hematocrit was 44.9. Since he began using a CPAP machine after his overnight sleep study, Cedric is sleeping better and has much more energy.

Challenges and Next Steps

Cedric, who has a family history of obesity, thought he was making improvements in his lifestyle and taking good care of himself. In reality, he was traveling a lot and it was hard for him to stay on any sort of regular schedule with regard to exercise and nutrition.

The Takeaways

Cedric wanted to set realistic goals and stick to them. Small improvements are better than none. If you know you can't eat well one week, make sure you eat well in the surrounding weeks. If you know you will be traveling and won't be able to get to a gym, find a trainer to help you set up a routine that you can implement anywhere. Be sure to sustain balance in the complete blood count (CBC) values by eating a wide variety of vegetables and adding supplements, especially if your lab indicates deficiencies in vitamin B. With low iron, most men will need to get a specialist for a colonoscopy, though hemorrhoids can also be an underlying reason for losing blood.

IMPROVING THE FILTRATION SYSTEM: LIVER FUNCTION

JENSEN D. was like many of our men—he had no idea he was diabetic. He just knew he was gaining weight and felt lousy most of the time. Jensen's lab tests revealed that he had elevated levels of ALT and SGPT, two biomarkers of liver malfunction. If your levels are elevated, you may want to schedule a liver ultrasound and check your blood for any viral infections, like mononucleosis, Epstein-Barr virus, or hepatitis.

Jensen's ultrasound showed he had fatty liver deposits, which are commonly found along with diabetes. This happen when diabetes has gone unchecked and has begun to damage the liver; it also occurs with obesity and high cholesterol. Jensen unfortunately had all three issues.

Problems

- Fatty liver deposits, liver function problems

- Diabetic and didn't know it. Hemoglobin A1c was high at 6.7 percent, and his fasting glucose and insulin levels were elevated as well.

- Low testosterone

- Low libido and marital strife

Corrections

After scheduling him for a 2-hour glucose tolerance test, which gave me a more in-depth picture about how his body was processing carbs, I started him on metformin and Victoza. I recommended that Jensen eat smaller portions more often and add more protein to each meal, especially breakfast. I suggested that he reduce his carb intake to 10 grams per meal.

I also started him on:

- Crestor, when his particle testing from Berkeley HeartLab showed elevated bad LDL small particles

- Testosterone injections to correct the finding of low T

- DHEA (precursor to testosterone), vitamin D_3, melatonin (for sleep), CoQ10 (taken with the Crestor, it helps to prevent body aches), alpha-lipoic acid, glucosamine chondroitin and MSM (for arthritis), omegas, baby aspirin, and juice powders, too.

Improvements

Within a year, Jensen's ALT and SGPT levels had come down within acceptable range and his fasting insulin was undetectable. His testosterone levels also improved. Still, his hemoglobin A1c was high at 6.3 percent, and his fasting glucose was elevated at 103 mg/dL. This was partly due to Jensen's stressful life and his inability to make any changes in the face of his current circumstances.

Challenges and Next Steps

Once Jensen's testosterone levels rebounded, I saw an increase in his estradiol, a by-product of testosterone via aromatase. This was not surprising, as Jensen was overweight, and aromatase is particularly abundant in fat. I prescribed anastrozole (Arimidex) to prevent the conversion of testosterone to estrogen. As Jensen lost weight and his body adjusted to the higher testosterone levels, I was able to take him off the Arimidex.

Jensen had a very difficult home life. His wife constantly undermined his efforts to get in shape and take time for himself. Because he wasn't consistent with implementing changes to his diet, Jensen's carb metabolism remained abnormal. Not surprisingly, too, despite improved testosterone levels, he suffered from low libido, problems with sexual function, and was decidedly unhappy.

The Takeaways

If your lab results show your liver biomarkers ALT and SGPT are elevated like Jensen's, you may want to consider getting advanced liver function testing, which may include an ultrasound or a liver biopsy. Fatty liver deposits can be detected with an ultrasound, and if you've got them, you've likely got a problem with your carbohydrate metabolism— how you're converting food into fuel. In addition to lifestyle changes that include sleep, food, fitness, and stress, you'll need medication to manage your glucose and insulin.

If hepatitis C, cancer, mononucleosis, or some other infection or virus that would impair liver function is suspected, there are a few steps you'll have to take. First, your doctor will have to find out your viral load by doing a liver biopsy. Next, he or she will have to check for evidence of cirrhosis. Treatment options will range depending on your diagnosis.

HOW DO YOU GET STARTED?

Overall there's a common theme here: Almost every man coming into my office has a compromised hormonal panel. This is common and likely the main reason for the decline in metabolism that starts at around age 40. These declines are reversible. It's about knowing hormone levels, free testosterone especially, and then examining these numbers in relation to your carbohydrate metabolism biomarkers, kidney and liver biomarkers, lipids, complete blood count (CBC), and inflammatory markers. Gathering these stats, along with your personal health metrics, will allow you to know which interventions may help jump-start your system and increase your health span. Sometimes it's challenging if you don't have a baseline to compare where you are now to where you were in your twenties. You can still take action today by tracking your progress through your labs and lifestyle improvements.

The men in these stories have turned around many disorders of aging and are somewhere along their own path to optimal health. It's your turn to take the first steps toward maximizing your health span. After all, while excellent health may be a great destination, it is also a highway with endless exits that are the results of choices you make daily.

Where does your road map take you? Detours and roadwork—holidays, travel, the flu, falling off the wagon—are to be expected. Those orange cones are annoying, but they sure do tell you something too. They're warning signs. Take opportunities to step back, readjust and check your compass and your map. How many times would the GPS have led you to the wrong destination had you not looked at a map before you left?

There is an old Marine saying, known as the Seven P's: Prior proper preparation prevents piss-poor performance. Peyton Manning, who was never a Marine but who many believe will go down as one of the greatest quarterbacks to ever play in the NFL, is also one of the most prepared. To get his teammates, especially the wide receivers, on the same page, he has them first look at the playbook from an "airplane view." From the first days of organized team activity through the team's time at training camp, Manning and his offense begin to zoom in on the playbook, getting into further detail. Toward the end of the preseason, everything is examined through a microscope. While this process takes but a few months in the NFL, these players have been training much of their lives and also have many seasons under their belts.

Thus, when it comes to your health, I would zoom in or out according to your distant and recent history to come up with your playbook for optimizing health span. During this first go-around, you may need to look at your map from the sky—seeing the forest, not the trees—thinking of the next year of your life as your current season.

Keeping the full picture in mind, you'll want to set up a list of steps that will deal with your key priorities. After you get everything in order in terms of collecting your personal metrics, it's your efforts that count. By putting in the time (remember, Joe Nicolla said at the beginning of the chapter that it can be done in about 4 hours a week) and achieving metabolic balance and consistency, you'll be able to optimize your health.

SETTING GOALS

The law of inertia says: A body at rest will stay at rest unless acted upon by an outside force. By the same token, a body in motion will stay in motion unless it collides with some sort of roadblock. If you've been active for a long time, then what has kept you going? What will keep you going? If you have not been exercising, eating right, or keeping yourself healthy, what has been standing in your way? Inspiration to shape up is all around you, if you choose to see it. Let's take a step back and look at the bigger picture of your life. Start with the information you use to introduce yourself. Take a pencil and fill in the blanks:

I'm ____ years old. My career is _____, which requires ____ to ____ hours per week of my time.

Maybe you have a family:

_____ (significant other's name) and I have been together _____ years. During this time, we have traveled to _____ and done _____ (number, description of activities). I have _____ kids, who are _____, _____, _____, _____, _____ years of age. Their names are _____, _____, _____, _____, _____. They _____, _____, _____ (go to school, participate in extracurricular activities, play sports, etc.). We have extended family in the following places _____, _____, _____ whom we see _____ times per _____.

Now, add up the number of hours that you work and perform other obligations each week from Monday to Friday. Subtract that from 120. (If you often find yourself working weekends as well, use 168 as your total.) Take away an additional 40 hours from that to allot for the suggested 8 hours of sleep you're supposed to get each day. With that, you'll have your excess number of hours per week: _____. Let's formulate how much of that time you can spend getting yourself to a stronger, more vibrant place in one year. First, you need to set goals. Set work, stress, and everything else aside for a moment.

A year from now, I would like to _____, _____, _____, *and* _____. Answers could range from taking that trip you always wanted to do or getting back on that surfboard for the first time since your kids were born. Maybe you've wanted to learn how to play guitar, drop 20 pounds, and have enough stamina to coach your kids' soccer games. Or perhaps you're a former collegiate athlete looking for a new challenge and you're itching to participate in a triathlon and have enough energy left over to take on the new China account at work.

Let's look at some concrete goals you can make now to help you get there.

Six months from now, I would like to _____, _____, _____, *and* _____. Answers could include a 10- to 20-pound total shift in body composition (gaining one pound of muscle is +1; losing a pound of fat is also +1); running a 5-K race, maybe for charity; fitting into some old clothes you haven't been able to wear in a while (your favorite jeans, perhaps); or showing off your body at a family or school reunion.

Two months from now, I will _____, _____, _____, *and* _____. These answers could be: Increase flexibility, strength, and/or endurance; wake up with more energy, ready to take on the day; get better rest; improve my sex life.

This week, I will _____, _____ *and* _____. Good answers would be: Sign up for the gym (assuming you're cleared to exercise by your doctor); look up an educated, experienced, and reputable personal trainer; buy healthy groceries; figure out how to eat healthy meals during an upcoming week of meetings and dinners out with colleagues, clients, or family.

Today, I will _____, _____ *and* _____. Answers could be: Go for a walk; eat a healthier dinner than usual; identify people in your life who will cheer you on—this could be friends, family, colleagues at the office, people in the community.

POINTING TOWARD THE FUTURE

The body is still a mystery, like it or not. It's a magical thing. We're so complex, still mostly unknown. If you observe carefully and pay attention to your personal health metrics, you will begin to appreciate patterns and responses within yourself and your system. Your health can be maintained and restored if you are aware of your function and makeup.

"Always try and be better," Joe said in reference to successful people at the very beginning of this chapter. Don't try. Be better.

CHAPTER 12

THE FUTURE OF MEDICINE, TODAY

Practice the simple, time-honored concepts of good health and embrace the technology of Precision Medicine to lengthen your health span

My lifestyle didn't change. I think some people misinterpret lifestyle for the way you live. I get up in the morning, I work out, I eat, I go to work, I go to restaurants every night. That didn't change. What I did was change the ingredients that made the recipe up for my lifestyle. The ingredients had been butter and cream and all that stuff, and then they were different nutrients. I also didn't eat as much. I still made the cake every day, but the way I made the cake and the way I ate the cake changed. It's important to make that distinction because your lifestyle doesn't change. You can't tell me: Don't work 10 hours or 15 hours a day. That's just the way it is. Lots of people will say: I don't have time to work out because I do this and I travel and all that kind of stuff. I hear that all the time and that's crap. It's just an excuse for not changing what you do. And I find most people do that. The truth is, as with anything in life, if you want to do it, you have purpose. First comes purpose and then comes the passion. Passion to me is purpose on steroids. You really have to be excited about your purpose and then you get passionate.

—JOE PLUMERI, 70, former chairman and CEO of Willis Group Holdings

The fact is, you probably give more attention to your car's health than you give to your own. That won't cut it. If your goal is to work 60 hours, play 18 holes of golf as well as a set of singles tennis, and spend a great day hiking in the mountains with your family during the weekend, then you need to plan for that just as you would outfit a race car with the appropriate tools and parts. What kind of tires do you need? What kind of fuel will yield extreme performance? What kind of headlights will help you see the farthest down the road? Moreover, what can you do to maximize your performance for as long as possible?

Your health is an ongoing process. So if you desire to be like a high-performance car, you need to know your goals and have the tools to track them over time. You need to be able to diagnose what you have today and predict obstacles to your future well-being. And you may need to augment what you currently have in order to find your sweet spot.

Disorders of aging are mostly preventable and reversible. Here's what you need to remember in the process of transforming your sedan into a race car:

1. Focus on yourself and the specifics, where you are now and where you want to go. Change happens on a cellular level on a scale of nanoseconds. Make observations about where you are now and compare it to how you felt in the past. Know that if you're over 40, you may have a compromised hormone picture, with low testosterone contributing to your lack of energy, mental fogginess, low libido, as well as various disorders of aging.

2. Capture your history, and not only your past medical history, but also that of your family members. Also, pay attention to the lifestyle choices you're making with regard to sleep, stress, sex, food, and fitness. Take ownership of the factors within your control, and make decisions that will help you increase your health span.

3. Get all the data you need so that you can begin to invest in yourself and make changes. There is no normal, no average. There is only what's right for your individual situation. Get your baseline stats. If you don't have lab results from your twenties, get the tests you need now and monitor them over intervals of 3, 4, and 6 months, based on the rate you opt to change. The more you do, the faster you move, the earlier you'll want to measure. Usually 10 to 12 weeks is the shortest interval to assess significant differences. Tracking your personal health metrics over time will show you what you're doing well and where you may need improvement.

4. Each system in the body impacts all others. You can't isolate an organ for treatment. It's difficult to increase your health span without taking your whole system into account.

5. There are no absolutes in medicine, and each individual is unique based on his genetics and experience, and how those two interact (more on that a bit later). It follows then that no two paths to optimizing health look exactly the same.

6. Develop a partnership with your doctor. Find someone who's knowledgeable, open-minded, and willing to think about prevention instead of intervention. Together you will be able to explore new ideas and new ways of working together.

7. Nobody can do the work for you. You need to be an active participant in maximizing your health span.

ON THE HORIZON

The technology and science of Precision Medicine are advancing at a rapid pace, offering new tools every day for gathering a more detailed understanding of what's happening in the human body at genetic, cellular, and molecular levels.

Larry Smarr, an astrophysicist-turned-computer-whiz, is one of the foremost self-quantifiers. He became obsessed with what he puts in his body, and more importantly, to him at least, what comes out. (He's particularly fastidious about analyzing his stool.) The *Atlantic* magazine ran a cover story in summer 2012 showing Smarr's progress on quantifying himself, a quest that started with wanting to lose weight and shifted toward overall health after he was diagnosed with Crohn's disease. He is constantly adding to his own personal metrics with countless data points about every aspect of his physiology. Ever optimistic, Smarr believes that with technology advancing at the pace it's at today, computers will be able to create a map of our insides, and not just a generalized map, but one specific to you and another unique to me. We're both talking about Precision Medicine (albeit in slightly different ways); our shared belief being that it will be the medicine of the future sooner rather than later.

Although medicine has come a long way in the past century, so much about your body is still an enigma, even with 21st-century advances in basic and clinical research. The medicine of the future will bring us opportunities to work synergistically to repair damage and prevent disease at much subtler levels and long before the trouble manifests in a major organ. In several places around the world, these interventions are already happening. I'm implementing many of them in my practice to chart a more precise path for each individual.

I apply three categories of interventional and diagnostic tools that aren't widely used yet. These are some of the recently developed methods that offer tremendous usefulness in predicting, discovering, and reversing disorders of aging:

1. **Genetics and epigenetics.** Genetic testing is undergoing a revolution, thanks to work done in the field of epigenetics, which is the study of how your genes interact with your environment based on a host of factors that can be either positive or negative.

2. **DNA repair and telomere length.** We now have the ability to detect and repair the damage to our DNA that accompanies aging. Indirectly, it is possible to prevent the shortening and damage of the protective ends of our chromosomes, called the telomeres, which leads to disease. And directly, reactivating the switch to reverse the DNA damage has become a reality.

3. **Controlling inflammation.** New tools such as the EndoPAT test give us a better understanding of the relationship between arterial inflammation and the disorders of aging, leading us to identify and address changes that are happening beneath the surface sooner than we may have otherwise, and in time to prevent disease.

Let's look more closely at how each of these cutting-edge tools is changing medicine today.

GENETICS AND EPIGENETICS

Interest in genetic testing is booming, and why not? A simple blood draw or cheek swab can reveal aspects about your DNA that may put your mind at ease or help you prepare to face your future. And as you saw in Chapter 10, genetic screening can even predict your responsiveness to a specific drug for depression, an infection, or cancer. It also can tell you if you're at greater risk for developing atrial fibrillation or a select neurological disorder. We're only just beginning to appreciate its many practical applications.

Genetic testing is especially beneficial for people who are adopted or have gaping holes in their knowledge of family history. One such patient of mine who is adopted comes to mind. When we first met, he knew little of his biological makeup. Genetic testing showed that he was at extremely high risk for developing prostate cancer, so I implemented safeguards to be proactive years ahead of the possible emergence of disease. Knowing a patient's genetic risk allows me to chart a course with that individual that either avoids the issue entirely, or converts it into a more manageable alternative that allows me to monitor the advances in the field that might yield a solution for him.

In fact, today's medicine is using genetic information to make changes in fetuses. A September 2006 article in the *New York Times* reported that Chad Kingsbury, who lost his mother, grandfather, and two uncles to colon cancer, was determined not to pass that genetic risk on to his children. He preselected sperm that didn't carry the genetic marker for colon cancer so that his unborn child wouldn't be dealt the same hand. The more we learn about genetics, the more we may be able to trade in our 2 and 7 for a pair of aces.

Consider this: If you carried a gene for an incurable disease, would you want to know? A December 2012 CBS News poll found that 58 percent of Americans would want to learn if they had a disease that couldn't be cured.

My patient Wade B. did not initially share the majority view. Raised by his stepfather, Wade didn't know much about his biological father. When he came to me, he had a number of disorders including bipolar depression, obesity, diabetes, and high cholesterol.

Wade's main concern was whether he was likely to develop early-onset Alzheimer's, which typically emerges before age 65 and cannot be altered as effectively with changes in lifestyle. This rare, aggressive form

Genetic Screening for Alzheimer's

Research shows that we can genetically screen people in their thirties or forties to detect earlier onset of Alzheimer's disease. By screening early, we can come up with treatments that might have a better chance of working.

According to the Alzheimer's Association, the disease affects about 13 percent of Americans age 65 and older, nearly 50 percent of those 85 or older. A study reported in *Journal Watch Neurology* shows that Alzheimer's is likely being diagnosed too late: up to 2 decades after the biological process has begun. If the disease starts 20 years before it manifests, then, says the study, it's no surprise that we haven't figured out an effective way to treat it.

The solution might lie in genetic screening for people without symptoms as young as 30 or 40 to establish risk. This is why knowing family history can be important—it can uncover red flags and indicate a direction for further testing. If you don't know your family history, genetic testing is certainly an alternative.

of Alzheimer's, which typically affects only 5 percent of people with Alzheimer's disease, is linked to three genes—APP, PSEN1, and PSEN2. Wade decided he wanted to know if he had a genetic mutation in one of those genes.

Once Wade's DNA sample had been drawn, however, he called the office many times telling me he was having second thoughts; he had thought he wanted to know, but now he wasn't so sure. How would the results influence the rest of his life? Because of his executive role at his company, would he have to acknowledge the results publicly? How would the results impact him and his professional life once any condition was reported to insurers? Would fears of the disease affect his day-to-day personal life? In Wade's case, the story turned out fine. He didn't test positive for the Alzheimer's mutation. He was relieved for himself and for his children. It's tough to say how he would have felt had the results not been negative. Early-onset Alzheimer's has no cure. Yet earlier detection gives people the chance to put plans in place and explore therapeutic interventions that might delay onset of symptoms.

But here's an important point: In many cases, genetics are not destiny. Changes in lifestyle may alter your risk of developing disease. Remember Wayne Hickory from Chapter 7? Once he received his results that showed that he had a single mutation on the 9p21 gene, thereby increasing his cardiovascular risk by nearly 50 percent, he began to eat extra helpings of raw fruits and vegetables. This simple lifestyle change has been shown to neutralize cardiovascular risk, possibly reducing it to nearly zero.

Imagine you had the kind of risk Wayne carries and knew you could take steps to reverse that risk. Would you switch up your diet? If you knew that your children carried the gene, and that the time to have a major impact on health is during childhood and adolescence, would you encourage a similar approach to diet and nutrition in your family life? Actually, I think the better question is: Why not?

Welcome to the emerging field of epigenetics. Data have shown that life experiences and exposure may change the very nature of your health and your genes.

You can see the impact of epigenetics in identical twins, whom scientists once believed were completely the same with regard to their genes. *National Geographic* reported on this emerging field in a January 2012 article that discussed twin boys, both born with autism. One of the brothers was reading and using an iPad by the age of 8, while the other spoke only a few words and expressed himself by flapping his hands. The twin who was less functional had a series of infections during his first year of life. Those infections probably impacted his development.

I am an identical twin myself. My sister Harriet is a dermatologist in Wyomissing, Pennsylvania. Even though we look alike and are both doctors, our personalities are distinct. We have different tastes. I will eat sushi at every opportunity, whereas my sister dislikes fish, especially sushi. Our blood work differs, too. We have a couple of genetic variations that are not identical. How could that happen?

Identical twins diverge in their identicalness from the moment the cells divide after fertilization and then implant at different places in the womb; their nourishment will even be distinct, by virtue of placement in the womb. As my sister and I grew up, we had unique experiences, all of which altered the nature of who we were on every level, including our genes. The same set of genes is expressed in different ways. One sibling, for example, develops metabolic syndrome with diabetes, obesity, and high cholesterol while the other does not, yet they both carry the gene. Scientists explained this as variable "penetrance"; simply stated, the gene expressed itself or it didn't. We really didn't have a better explanation.

In the very recent past, 80 percent or so of the DNA spirals were considered "junk" genes, inactive. This notion has been completely abandoned, for good reason—it never really made sense. Why would we contain worthless DNA tightly wound up in such complex systems that we know so little about? The data published by the ENCODE project in the September 2012 issue of *Nature* were proof that it is becoming increasingly clear just how much more there is to learn as we delve further in the human genome.

Until recently, DNA genes were thought to be active if they controlled the production of proteins within our system. Recall from high school biology that DNA can either halt or promote protein production via messenger RNA. What was unknown is that those classic spirals contain a system of switches of their own, and those switches can either activate or deactivate the genes themselves, similar to turning a light on and off. Various triggers may induce the click. In essence, the DNA, protein producing in conjunction with the switches that modify them, are likely responsible for the way you operate and the quality of function you have, such as whether or not you will have a heart attack or arthritis. In effect, we all carry a regulation system within the very DNA that decides how to behave and is highly influenced by our own decisions. It is already clear that cells have to predetermine where, when, and how each will do what—a heart cell works in the heart, while the bone cell or testes cell acts accordingly as well. Can cell behavior be altered, too? Perhaps the switch turns off certain DNA, depending on your lifestyle, which could explain how upping the intake of raw fruits and veggies might switch off the 9p21 SNP on Wayne Hickory's genes.

Each of us can choose not to become victims of our genes and internal aging, held hostage to switches that might pay attention if only you adjust what you eat or optimize your protein intake. Maybe we can pull one over on Mother Nature? I think so, and clearly my patients see it happen as they modify aspects of their behavior. Yet much still needs to be explored.

Does this model converge with the newer concept of epigenetics? Of course. We can no longer shrug our shoulders and blame our parents for passing down those less than desirable genes. We can do something about them!

In the past, scientific research has been shaped by the binary paradigm of nurture versus nature. With epigenetics, we come to find that life is not necessarily a battle between nurture and nature but rather a more complex interplay: Nurture plus nature, plus the innumerable events and choices, that moment by moment, shape who you are and what you do. Each time you add a variable, the equation is not simply 1 + 1 + 1—it's a logarithmic factor with nearly incalculable variations and permutations. You are a complex being, the result of the somewhat unpredictable combination of countless factors. That complexity goes all the way down to the molecular instructions for the expression of your genes: your DNA.

DNA AND TELOMERES

The field of epigenetics studies how lifestyle, exposure, and environment, taken together, can impact your genetics. Taking a closer look at your DNA adds another layer of complexity to the equation. Telomeres are the tips of your DNA, and like the caps on shoelaces, they unravel and shorten with replication. We've gained insight into the aging process by studying them.

In the last couple of decades, it's been shown that telomeres are a kind of life-length predictor. Originally looking at a single-celled pond-dwelling organism called a *Tetrahymena,* geneticists discovered that there are a set number of replications DNA can make before the ends of the telomeres begin to fray and deteriorate. When this happens, you become more susceptible to disease.

Scientists are now starting to look at the percentage of short telomeres people have relative to others, stratifying by age and gender. It's thought that this percentage may be a predictor for your biological age. If you have an excessive percentage of short telomeres, your chronological age may be 50, but your biological age may be closer to 70.

This simple blood test to measure telomere length is performed only at the University of Madrid by a company called Life Length, founded by Maria Blasco, PhD. The company's database is still evolving, yet investigation into telomeres is booming and will certainly be part of your future.

In fact, telomere research has already had an impact on a specific but rather diverse group of people. The National Institutes of Health reports that it's highly common to contract cytomegalovirus, often a mild case, during your life and sometime before age 40. Reports estimate that 50 to 80 percent of adults have been exposed. The symptoms can mimic a ferocious cold, and the virus can cause fatigue and abnormal results in liver function tests. Once you've had the virus, you develop antibodies to it, which show up in a blood test. It appears that exposure to cytomegalovirus compromises the immune system in some way, so that your immune function may not be as robust as somebody who never had the virus. A study found that telomeres were shortened in a group of people who had cytomegalovirus. In contrast, however, to non-exposed individuals, the first group responded in a shorter period of time to a supplement that lengthens telomeres.

This preliminary research indicates there may be a way to reverse the telomere damage from cytomegalovirus, and I have begun to use that same supplement that proactively elongates telomeres, even those that have been shortened over time. Cultivated from a high-density root of the herb astragalus, the supplement promotes telomerase activation. Traditional Chinese medicine has made use of astragalus for centuries, and now Western medicine is recognizing its benefits.

Average telomere length, regardless of whether telomeres were initially defined as short, medium, or long, appears to increase across the board when people exposed to the cytomegalovirus use astragalus. Immune system function seems to improve over time as well. Of course, more research is needed, and the results will have to be replicated in larger populations; nevertheless, early results are promising.

I've started several patients on TA-65, which is a brand of astragalus available from T.A. Sciences. (*Note:* I receive no compensation from T.A. Sciences.) My overall data is yet to be published, but I'm getting better than expected results from my patients, likely because they are doing so many things to improve their well-being besides using TA-65. Once my patients reach their sweet spot, many of them develop strength, endurance, and health approximating that of a 30-year-old. As such, their response to TA-65 may be heightened. A preliminary evaluation of the individuals who've been on TA-65 for at least 1 to 2 years reveals a significant increase in average telomere length. While the lengthening effect wasn't observed in all patients, there was a net increase in the group. Typically, my patients showed a response within 12 months, and I was no exception.

I tried TA-65 first before I introduced it to my patients. Given my background in clinical research, I like to test supplements out on myself before I make the decision to offer them to patients. If possible, I also prefer to change one variable at a time while keeping everything else the same, the idea being to create as controlled an environment as possible. That way, whatever differences I notice are more likely to be attributed to the variable in question—in this case, the TA-65.

In late 2009, I started taking TA-65. I had heard it helped improve vision, but I didn't give it much thought with regard to my own situation. (I wear contact lenses to correct for nearsightedness, although I need reading glasses to see small print.) When I went to my ophthalmologist, who had been examining my eyes for 20 years at Yale, he was surprised by what he found.

"Okay, Florence," he said. "What have you been up to now? Your eyes have changed, and they shouldn't have." In that instant, it occurred to me that I had stopped using the reading glasses stashed in every purse, drawer, and lab coat. I don't know exactly when I stopped, I only knew that now I wasn't using them at all. My environment hadn't changed, nothing else about my health had changed, yet I no longer needed them.

Jump to September 2012. A Yale medical school classmate referred me to an optometrist in New York who, unlike my ophthalmologist back in New Haven, Connecticut, had no knowledge of me, my medical history, or my lifestyle. My chief complaint during the 2012 visit was that I often needed to take off my glasses to read because things appeared to be too magnified. When he measured my eyes, he was shocked to find that, indeed, my prescription was too strong and my contacts needed to be refitted. His explanation was that the Yale ophthalmologist had no idea how to measure the lens correctly. I knew that my eyes had continued to improve over time. It was only by getting my records and comparing them to the current findings that my optometrist was able to see that difference. There are other anecdotal stories from individuals with clinical improvements (in skin, hair, stamina, energy), though these reports are not yet published in the peer-reviewed scientific literature.

Certainly, astragalus and its effect on telomere lengthening is something that warrants further exploration. There appears to be few downsides to taking it, although there is some concern that if you activate telomerase, you may activate cancer cells. Data in mice and rats show that this hasn't occurred. In fact, short telomeres are alleged to trigger cancer in a rodent model. As with anything new, proceed with caution. If you are interested, discuss the supplement in depth with your health advisors and clinicians. An additional concern is cost. Right now TA-65 and other brands on the market are very expensive, ranging from $200 to $600 for 1 to 2 months, depending on the number of caps taken daily. Expect that price to drop within the next 10 years as the area of genetics and DNA sequencing grows.

THE ENDOPAT TEST: DETECTING INFLAMMATION RELATED TO ARTERIAL FUNCTION

Nick E. had had a heart attack before he was referred to me. The visit to the hospital, complete with sirens and gurney, came as a bit of a surprise to him because his lab tests had showed that his total cholesterol levels were good. (Remember, cholesterol is a marker that predicts heart disease.) Even Nick's LDL was okay. Maybe it was inching toward the upper limits of what I consider acceptable, yet it was still within range. His doctors told him not to be worried.

Nick isn't an anomaly. You already know that many people who have cholesterol levels considered within range will have a heart attack or stroke. In fact, perhaps as many as 75 percent of individuals hospitalized with a heart attack have *normal* cholesterol. There are other factors we need to take into account.

Inflammation is a critical one. I believe it's the common denominator to disease. Inflammation signifies damage, injury, or change in the body. Our bodies are producing free radicals constantly, whether it's from eating or working out, activities that are critical to existence. These free radicals ping around our system, damaging our DNA and causing inflammation. Inflammation at a cellular level may prevent you from combating disease.

So how do you get your arms around addressing these tiny, invisible, cellular issues?

Your lab results, which will measure inflammatory markers c-CRP and homocysteine, are a good start. They offer broad diagnostic insight because they speak to the total health of your body, yet they don't show how inflammation directly impacts function. The results of an EndoPAT test will.

In the last 2 years, my practice has added the EndoPAT to our series of diagnostic tests. Done in the office, the EndoPAT test helps me measure how the arteries are functioning at a cellular level, giving us details about the status of your circulatory system that we can't get from a blood sample. The EndoPAT machine is able to detect deteriorating function in the vascular system, just like cardiac catheterizations, CAT scans of the heart vessels, or even carotid ultrasounds. Yet the EndoPAT is noninvasive, takes only about 20 minutes to complete, and is covered by most insurance plans.

You've heard me mention endothelium in conjunction with c-CRP. It lines the heart vessels as well as all the arteries in your body, and it's critical in facilitating the movement of blood throughout your body. As you get older, blood vessels get stiffer. If there's inflammation in the endothelium, it means the vessels won't rebound as effectively as they should, impairing circulation due to increased resistance (stiffer pipes), leading to a decline in heart function.

Remember, too, nitric oxide is critical for endothelial function, as it promotes vasodilation and bloodflow. When there's dysfunction on the level of the endothelium, not enough nitric oxide is produced, which affects not only cardiovascular function but also sexual performance.

With the EndoPAT, I can determine inflammation in the endothelium by looking at the responsiveness of those vessels. First, the bloodflow in your brachial artery is obstructed for 5 minutes, like getting your blood pressure taken, except the cuff stays tight longer, for about 15 minutes. When the cuff is removed, the EndoPAT device measures how quickly the vessels allow blood to flow back into the arm. I like to see the measurement (known as the reactive hyperemia index, or RHI) above 2, with a goal of 2.8 for optimal health. If your number is lower than 2, inflammation in your blood vessels may be a big enough problem to cause erectile dysfunction, heart attacks, or strokes. By knowing your EndoPAT score and combining it with other inflammatory markers, I can get a much better indication of your risk for disease, and I can target this trigger for disease with all the weapons in the arsenal of this book.

OPTIMIZING HEALTH SPAN: BEYOND GENETICS

What I've thought was predestined about health turns out to be within our own control. Genetic patterns don't absolutely predict metabolism, health span, or the emergence of disease. James Markham, for example, is 83. According to a June 2012 Bloomberg article, his four siblings died of cancer, heart disease, and emphysema by the age of 62. Markham himself remembers being sick only once: He had a chest cold 50 years prior. Scientists are studying his genes, along with those of more than 1,000 healthy elderly people, to find out what they may have in their genome sequencing that's keeping them from succumbing to the disorders of aging. They carry about the same percentage of genes for disorders of aging as the rest of the population, yet they're not developing the diseases.

From his family history, you would have thought the quality of Markham's health span would be dismal. On the surface, he wasn't dealt a great genetic hand—and he most likely carries overlapping genes for the disorders of aging carried by his siblings. An elusive, indefinable component—whether it was optimism, a certain fight in his personality, or his daily decisions about what he consumed and how he lived—was perhaps altering how his genes were being expressed. Genetics tells you what genes you have. Epigenetics tells you how your genes have been turned on or off by how you live. But it may be the truly intangible that makes the biggest difference of all.

The book *The Blue Zones* and an October 2012 *New York Times* article about the Greek island of Ikaria, 30 miles off the coast of Turkey, have presented similar information on why certain people are living considerably longer with enviable health spans. A "blue zone" is a region of the world defined as a "longevity hotbed." People commonly lead active lives past the age of 100 years. Such is the case for the residents of Ikaria. They have the same genetic material as those from neighboring islands, they eat a similar diet, and the environment is nearly identical. Yet they are living longer and staying more alert than their neighbors. Something subtle and powerful is going on there. The factors that make the difference are about as non-technological as they could be.

The Ikarians are well-rested, sleeping long, and napping regularly. Everybody contributes to sustaining the community, and that includes keeping gardens to feed themselves. They eat what's inexpensive and accessible, which turns out to be healthy and delicious. They walk up and down a lot of hills every day to get where they need to go. They are rarely alone or lonely. Everyone knows what everybody else is doing, so there's no opportunity to commit a crime and get away with it. The workday ends with tea and wine with neighbors, and the weekends are devoted to worship and other activities with the Eastern Orthodox Church.

All of these practices—particularly community, sleep, moderate exercise, faith, and a sense of purpose—are the common elements of longevity and optimal health span. They are easy to engage in on Ikaria because everybody else is doing them. The same thing happens in other "blue zones." But when you live in a culture that is diametrically opposed to healthy habits, how do you achieve well-being? It works when you begin to experience the positive feedback from making one change at a time to your own life. It helps to surround yourself with like-minded people.

It's difficult for anyone but you to know where you need to start and what will work for you in creating the conditions for a robust health span. You're always going to be making adjustments. Think of trying to balance with your eyes closed, maybe even on one foot. You will feel your body making constant little adjustments to remain standing. Your foot will wobble. More weight shifts to the instep, and the next moment you're supporting yourself on the outer edge of your heel. Your abs may engage. Maybe you extend an arm out like a tightrope walker balancing on a high wire.

With your eyes closed, the vestibular system in your ears (those little hair cells) work hard to keep you upright. That missing sense of sight is analogous to what you might not know about yourself and what we still don't know in medicine. After more than 20 years of studying genetics, it's abundantly clear that there is much medical science needs to learn about the human body. I have limits in understanding how your system functions that keep me from being able to give you exact details for managing your well-being. Yet even though you may be in the dark, you can reach that equilibrium.

By putting together an approach that diversifies your choices and has you covering as many bases as you can, you're going to add active, healthy years to your life. These future assessments that look at genetics and epigenetics, telomere length and arterial function will help fine-tune your balance. The trick is to start small and keep going.

Florence Comite has the perfect balance between the past and the future. She's a cautiously optimistic open-minded skeptic. While she's practicing a medicine of the future, she's conservative too. Everything she does is 100 percent based in science.

—BRUCE WENIG, MD,
chair of the department of diagnostic pathology and laboratory medicine, Beth Israel Medical Center & St. Luke's-Roosevelt Hospitals

PRECISION MEDICINE

It's time to take the next step into the future. Medicine needs to undergo a metamorphosis in which we revive the heart and soul of the family doctor but also take advantage of the remarkable advances in technology that focus on individual quantification. It's time to take the next step into the future. What we need instead of body-part specialists is a new multidisciplinary field called Precision Medicine that trains physicians to be guides and advisors: Physicians who can, in partnership with each patient, analyze tests and personal health metrics to optimize health span. We need doctors who know our lives and hopes on such a level that they have the ability to guide us—in concert with our desires—on the best path to avoid disease.

We're at a turning point in our medical system. The current model can take you in different directions. You can continue on the road of being shuttled from the internist to the specialist to the hospitalist who steps in to manage your care when you are admitted to a hospital. Or you can hope to turn to a new kind of doctor, a physician advisor, in the emerging specialty of Precision Medicine, who consults with specialists and guides the process of care before disease manifests. This transition to Precision Medicine will take years to implement from the perspective of medical schools and training. Clearly, our current system of health care will exist until such time, likely decades, mainstream medicine adapts to accommodate to an individualized health-centric delivery system. The hospitalist, trauma surgeon, and other acute care interventionists will still be necessary as there will always be a need for critical care, accidents and injuries being unavoidable.

The Precision Medicine clinician integrates the knowledge of a traditional family doctor with the best of the new advancements on the horizon. This new type of advisor might know you for years; he or she might know your extended family and also your family history, allowing for more meaningful guidance to prevent your decline as the years progress.

If I had my dream come true, we would institute this Precision Medicine model and move from the disease-centric form of health care that's currently taught and practiced throughout our country to a health-centric model. Medicine would be about meaningful personal prevention, and it would center on the specifics of the individual. Gone would be the days when crisis or insurance determined the course of care. That change is would only be the beginning. I think that in the coming decades, we will usher in this new age of Precision Medicine—an age in which there will be a high degree of specificity. We will come to own our own health care via our personal health metrics.

I have already seen a major shift in the last 20 years; it was evident at Yale a decade ago when I was teaching 1st- and 2nd-year medical students how to take a medical history from patients. The focus shifted from the doctor to the patient; from talking to listening. It was about hearing what the patient had to say, letting him finish his thoughts instead of jumping in to direct the conversation to conclusions that may not be relevant to why the patient was there to see you. It's harder to sustain that mind-set and have patience when you're crazed from stamping out disease that's already reached a state of emergency; however, the results are much more rewarding for both patient and doctor.

Changing the way physicians receive information from patients is only part of the solution. Critically important is recognizing the need for doctors to exchange data, especially when several are treating the same patient. The exchange of information has to put the patient at the center of care, with doctors using a common language and sharing perspectives with one another. There should be a central depository of information.

My mother was in the hospital for a week in 2011. Four different highly rated specialists cared for her. She had severe abdominal pain along with a very high white blood cell count. Each one of those doctors had a different opinion about what was going on in her belly. No one could drive a consensus. After careful review with my sister and me, my mother was put on a course of antibiotics, due to the elevated blood count, and she improved within the week. Who is going to be that wise person who takes in all the variables and figures out the pros and cons in each direction? How do you get to the final decision?

Doctors need to have the time to exchange data because it's so easy to miscommunicate. It's equally difficult for patients to get all the information they need from doctors and process it in a way that makes sense to them, free of medical jargon. Electronic medical records and systems might allow for a more ready exchange of data, organizing information in such a way that it delivers what you need to move forward and increase your health span. Precision Medicine will make the difference.

You've heard my patient Eran speak several times in the book. He's a physical therapist who often treats patients in a nursing home, a place where people of the Greatest Generation are going to die. It's often a long and miserable deterioration. And now we baby boomers struggle simultaneously with the health and care of our parents as well as our own. What will your health future look like?

I hope that after reading this book, you now have a different perspective. You can weigh the relevance of the information you're hearing or reading in the media against a deeper understanding of your own health. Does it apply to you? You know how to interpret evidence-based medicine better, too. You know that if you're an Asian man in California or Caucasian man living in New York, a study on a heart drug in Italian men living in Sicily might not apply to you. Genetics, epigenetics, your individual life experience, your lab data, all of it makes a difference.

What's important to remember is that our bodies are complex systems; we don't know what we don't know. How can we have all the answers when we don't even know the questions? Collecting the details over time and pairing them with our own observations will lead us toward healthy longevity.

I know that most of the future remains shrouded in mystery, and I'm leaving you with many questions when you were probably expecting answers. Then again, my inquisitive nature is something that was nurtured from the time I was very young. My father was on his own quest to live life to the fullest, way ahead of the mainstream medical world: jogging, dancing, swimming, traveling, always moving to stay healthy. I know my dad infused his love of learning, activity, and life into me, and, luckily, he and I passed these traits onto my two sons as well. Daily I get briefings from my boys about the latest in the medical news. We debate the pros and cons of certain food, exercises, medications, and supplements, and we discuss how medicine will be practiced 10 or 20 years from now. They started years ago, asking questions, always challenging, too, not satisfied with the status quo. Keeping up, staying ahead, there is no other option! For that, I am grateful. My father led the way, and my sons now add exponentially to the conversation and life's adventures. And here I am, hoping each day I will continue to transfer my father's wisdom—informed by my clinical experience, fueled by a foundation in academic medicine and research, and driven by my curiosity—to heal each one of my patients, and now, you.

Make your future be a healthy one.

ACKNOWLEDGMENTS

To my patients who have shared their stories, their pain, their accomplishments: I cherish your respect and your trust. Healing is in the process, and I am honored to partner with you on our journey.

Over the years a broad spectrum of professionals—teachers, physicians, and scientists—have taught me to heal others. I thank, from early years, my 6th grade teacher Herb Tillem, who treasured his students; Maxwell Cohen, my 10th grade marine biology teacher, who opened my eyes to the glistening universe of science; Earl Jagust, 12th grade English, who taught me how to transmit to others what I learned of this new universe; and Mary Jane Strcctt, 11th grade history and economics, who offered the global context for the study of all subjects. My clinical, academic, and research work has been conducted with some of the best minds at Brooklyn College of CUNY, Yale School of Medicine, Yale-New Haven Hospital, the National Institutes of Health (NIH), and various other hospitals and centers. Doctors Donald Hurst, Gerard Burrow, Aaron Lerner, Robert Gifford, Lynn Loriaux, Shirley McCarthy, Stanley Possick, Richard Hochberg, Nancy Angoff, Paul Barash, Alan DeCherney, Alan Yanoff, and, most recently, John Docherty have shaped the ways in which I interact with my patients. I've listened to and learned from the kindness, compassion, and dignity they show their patients, students, and colleagues.

The ComiteMD team has contributed mightily to this book. My office colleagues helped me artfully bring together medical knowledge and patient stories. Laura Hedli was instrumental in this task. Others who offered their expertise and support include Anita Beri, Tim Coyle, Moazah Ahmed, Steven Villagomez, Brent Halsey, Rex Chu, Susan Barrett, Jennifer Hankins, Melissa Levy, and Eran Kabakov. Each member of the

ComiteMD team, present and past, has left an indelible mark on me and our patients.

I thank family, friends, and colleagues who contributed to this book's creation. Nina Luban, high school confidante, sister-friend, was present at the birth of this book, and her insights were invaluable through the finishing touches. My twin, Harriet Comite, MD, and her partner, Alan Geltman, provided continual support. Barbara Blum and I have lived through thick and thin together. Lila Feinberg's assistance was appreciated. Bob Horton, Ed and Doris Zelinsky, Stuart and Joan Margolis formed a solid New Haven-based team. My niece, Laura Kaplan, offered honest editorial comments. The daughter of my heart and son-in-law, Jessica and Osher Kedar, always provided their unique support. My sons, Michael and Jonathan Cabin, faithfully read drafts, sent references, and cheered me on. Friend and colleague, Robert Peng, gave me tremendous positive Qi. Tom Dunkel, author of "Vigor Quest," in the *New York Times Magazine* on 01.15.10, set the stage for this book and has become a trusted colleague and friend. My partner Marc Klahr was a spirited sounding board throughout the writing process and chef par excellence at frequent, all-night editing, sessions.

I am grateful that my agent, Susan Ginsburg, saw the book's potential early on and stayed the course. I especially acknowledge my editor, Jeff Csatari at Rodale, who was always in my corner. Our collaborative interactions helped me develop the book. It was a difficult challenge to figure out how to convey information about an emerging field of medicine not yet formally taught in medical schools. New visions in medicine invariably arise amidst controversy; so I am grateful that Jeff was fascinated and engaged in the process.

I have tried to write this book in such a way that both the general reader and the physician will see the logic and the promise of Precision Medicine. I believe a major shift in health care is imminent and it involves, above all, patients acting in concert with physicians. This book is for those who want to take ownership of their health. You can ensure a better quality of life in the future through positive changes *right now*, to last your lifetime.

APPENDIX

PRECISION HEALTH QUESTIONNAIRE (PHQ)

This questionnaire has been adapted from the one I use in my practice to help patients collect their personal health metrics. It is designed to help patients gather as much information as they can about their personal medical history, family history, and lifestyle, all of which provide invaluable background data for your health. Keep this information in your medical files and share it with your physicians. You may also choose to go to the Web site KeepItUpTheBook.com, if you want to learn more about the steps you might implement once the initial data is collected and interpreted.

PERSONAL MEDICAL HISTORY

Provide the most recent date and results for the tests listed below.

Tests	Date	Results
Rectal exam		
Testing for blood in stool		
Prostate exam		
PSA		
Colonoscopy		
Resting EKG		
Stress EKG		
Stress echo		
Nuclear stress		
Chest x-ray		
Eye exam/eye pressures		

List any diagnostic procedures you have had. Provide the approximate date, reason for the procedure, and result.

_____

_____

_____

_____

_____

List all current medications, including dosage and frequency (prescription and/or over the counter) you take, and the reason why you are taking them.

_____

_____

_____

_____

_____

List all current supplements, including dosage and frequency (i.e., vitamins, herbs, nutritional supplements) you take, and the reasons why you are taking them. If it is easier, copy the labels and attach them to your completed questionnaire.

_____

_____

_____

_____

_____

_____

_____

Specific Medications

Do you use Viagra, Cialis, Levitra, or any other erectile enhancement drugs?
Have they helped you?
Do you use any other medication for sexual function?
Have you ever used testosterone, hCG, DHEA, or HGH?

Under the categories listed below, check the "yes" column if you are experiencing the listed symptom to a substantial or unusual degree.

Sexual Health   Yes

Difficulty attaining/maintaining an erection
  (or insufficient to maintain penetration)   ____
Lack of early morning erections   ____
Lack of desire/enjoyment   ____
Ejaculation causes pain   ____
Premature ejaculation   ____
Sexual drive underactive   ____
Sexual drive overactive   ____
Pain/coldness in penis   ____

Sexual Health *(cont.)*   **Yes**

Pain/coldness in testicles   ____

Swollen genitals   ____

Genital sores/lesions   ____

Swelling in groin   ____

Lump or mass in scrotum   ____

Varicose veins on scrotum   ____

Varicocele in testes   ____

Discharge from penis   ____

Past or present rash on penis   ____

Infertility   ____

Low sperm count   ____

Prostatitis (prostate infections)   ____

Hernia   ____

Jock itch   ____

Past or present sexually transmitted disease (specify)   ____

General Health   **Yes**

Frequent infections or illness   ____

Frequent colds   ____

Change in appetite   ____

Fatigue/weakness/loss of energy   ____

Lumps in neck, armpits, groin, or breast   ____

Broken bone(s) as an adult   ____

Heat/cold intolerance   ____

Other symptoms (please list)   ____

Skin and Hair   Yes

Dry/brittle and/or flaky hair   ____

Hair thinning or falling out   ____

Abnormal fingernails   ____

Toe or fingernail fungus   ____

History of skin disorder or skin condition   ____

Dry/brittle skin   ____

Acne   ____

Age spots   ____

Puffy, wrinkled skin   ____

Swelling/edema   ____

Change in skin color   ____

Dark circles under eyes   ____

Bumpy skin on face or back of arms   ____

Spider veins in nose and/or face   ____

Persistent rash/skin allergy   ____

Sores, boils, sties, lumps/lesions   ____

Slow or poor wound healing   ____

Excessive sweating or itching   ____

Flushing or hot flashes   ____

Bruise easily or excessively   ____

Allergies   Yes

Seasonal allergies   ____

Food allergies   ____

Latex or other environmental allergies   ____

Are you allergic to any drugs?   ____

Do you break out in hives?   ____

Eyes/Ears/Nose/Throat   **Yes**

Facial pain   _____

Change in vision   _____

Use of corrective lenses (glasses or contacts)   _____

Blurred or tunnel vision   _____

Double vision   _____

Eye pain/inflammation   _____

Hearing loss   _____

Ringing in ears   _____

Ear pain   _____

Balance problems   _____

Ear drainage   _____

Ear infections   _____

Nosebleeds   _____

Stuffy nose   _____

Nasal discharge   _____

Nasal/sinus infections   _____

History of nasal/facial injury   _____

Sore or bleeding gums   _____

Canker sores or cold sores   _____

Frequent sore throat/hoarseness   _____

Difficulty swallowing   _____

Cardiopulmonary   **Yes**

Pain in the left arm   _____

Chest pain at rest or while walking, running, or lifting weights   _____

Pain in chest or sides   _____

Frequent and recurring upper respiratory infections   _____

Fluid retention (e.g., swollen ankles, legs, etc.)   _____

Cannot tolerate much exercise   _____

Cardiopulmonary *(cont.)*   **Yes**

Difficulty breathing   ____

Chronic lung congestion   ____

Cough with sputum, with pain   ____

Wheezing   ____

History of asthma   ____

Heaviness in legs   ____

Calf muscle cramps while walking   ____

Heart pounds easily   ____

Heart misses beats or has extra beats   ____

Rapid heartbeat, fluttering   ____

Shortness of breath   ____

Heartburn after eating   ____

Exhaustion with minor exertion   ____

Erratic blood pressure   ____

High blood pressure   ____

Low blood pressure   ____

Breathing problems at night   ____

Difficulty lying flat   ____

History of tuberculosis   ____

History of heart attack   ____

History of heart murmur or irregularity   ____

History of pneumonia   ____

Metabolic   **Yes**

Certain foods cause ill feelings   ____

Difficulty gaining weight   ____

Difficulty losing weight   ____

Bad breath (no relief by brushing)   ____

Body odor (no relief by washing)   ____

Metabolic *(cont.)*   **Yes**

Total blood cholesterol above 200　　　　　　　　　　____

HDL cholesterol below 50　　　　　　　　　　　　　____

LDL cholesterol above 130　　　　　　　　　　　　____

Swollen (bulging) eyes　　　　　　　　　　　　　　____

History of thyroid disorder　　　　　　　　　　　　____

Cold hands and feet　　　　　　　　　　　　　　　____

Thinning or loss of outside portion of eyebrow　　　____

Gain weight easily　　　　　　　　　　　　　　　　____

Crave salt or salty foods　　　　　　　　　　　　　____

Blushing with no apparent cause　　　　　　　　　____

Feel tired or weak if meal is missed　　　　　　　　____

Wake up at night craving sweets　　　　　　　　　____

Need to drink caffeine to get going　　　　　　　　____

Feel tired 1 to 3 hours after eating　　　　　　　　____

Feel faint or weak　　　　　　　　　　　　　　　　____

Night sweats　　　　　　　　　　　　　　　　　　____

Increased thirst　　　　　　　　　　　　　　　　　____

Overweight　　　　　　　　　　　　　　　　　　____

Crave sweets (but eating sweets does not relieve symptoms)　____

Weight loss of more than 10 pounds in the last 6 months　____

Weight gain of more than 10 pounds in the last 6 months　____

Weight has fluctuated more than 10 pounds over last 5 years　____

Vascular   **Yes**

Swelling in the legs　　　　　　　　　　　　　　　____

Varicose veins　　　　　　　　　　　　　　　　　____

Coldness/discoloration in legs/feet　　　　　　　　____

History of blood clots　　　　　　　　　　　　　　____

Raynaud's syndrome　　　　　　　　　　　　　　____

Gastrointestinal/Urological Health   **Yes**

Lack of appetite   ____

Excessive appetite   ____

Abdominal pain   ____

Nausea/vomiting   ____

Heartburn/reflux   ____

Difficulty/pain with swallowing   ____

Dependency on antacids   ____

History of ulcers   ____

History of liver disorder   ____

Flatulence (gas) or bloating   ____

Gallbladder problems   ____

Irritable bowel syndrome   ____

Change in bowel habits   ____

Loss of bowel control   ____

Diarrhea   ____

Constipation (hard or effortful bowel movements)   ____

Hemorrhoids   ____

Blood in stool   ____

Change in stool (color/consistency)   ____

Rectal pain   ____

Frequent urination or scant urination/dribbling   ____

Burning during urination   ____

Loss of bladder control (including leaking)   ____

Excessive nighttime urination (specify number of times) ____

Blood in urine   ____

Frequent urinary tract infections   ____

Difficulty urinating or initiating stream   ____

Sense of urgency to urinate   ____

Gastrointestinal/Urological Health *(cont.)*   Yes

Retention—inability to urinate or empty bladder   ____

Excessive/decreased volume   ____

Abnormal color or odor of urine   ____

Kidney stones   ____

Neurological   Yes

Headaches   ____

Faintness   ____

Seizures/convulsions   ____

History of epilepsy   ____

Tremors/spasms   ____

Dizziness   ____

Tingling or numbness   ____

Balance problems   ____

Paralysis   ____

Muscle weakness   ____

Memory problems   ____

Loss of smell or taste   ____

Problems with attention and concentration   ____

History of accident/injury   ____

History of loss of consciousness   ____

History of stroke   ____

Joints/Muscles/Bones   Yes

Joint pain, swelling, or stiffness   ____

Arthritis   ____

Neck/back pain   ____

Limited/decreased range of motion   ____

Muscle tension or spasms   ____

Muscle weakness   ____

Muscle cramps   ____

Muscle pain   ____

History of gout   ____

History of rheumatic diseases   ____

History of injury/fractures   ____

Fibromyalgia   ____

Carpal tunnel syndrome   ____

Osteoporosis (decreased bone density)   ____

FAMILY HISTORY

Enter all the health information that you know about your immediate
family (you may wish to interview family members at family gatherings
with this chart in hand). In the left column, you'll find a comprehensive
list of medical disorders. In the right column, list names, ages, and relationship (i.e., father, maternal grandmother, paternal cousin, etc.) of
family members who are suffering from that illness or condition. If you
do not know of any family members with that particular illness or condition, write "none."

CONDITION	FAMILY MEMBER
Heart disease (heart attack, coronary artery disease, congestive heart failure)	
High blood pressure	
Abnormal EKG	
Cancer	
Anemia	
High cholesterol	
Diabetes	

CONDITION	FAMILY MEMBER
Endocrine gland disorders (thyroid, adrenal, pituitary)	
Weight control problems	
Lung disease (asthma, emphysema, bronchitis)	
Allergies	
Stomach/esophagus disorders (reflux, stricture, ulcers)	
Bowel disease (malabsorption, lactose intolerance, diverticulitis, Crohn's, colitis, irritable bowel syndrome)	
Liver disease (hepatitis, cirrhosis)	
Kidney disease (stones, infections, cysts)	
Bladder disease	
Autoimmune disease (lupus, rheumatoid arthritis)	
Arthritis	
Osteoporosis	
Neurological disorders (stroke, seizures, Parkinson's, Alzheimer's, multiple sclerosis)	
Migraine headaches	
Memory problems	
Sleep apnea/snoring	
Mental health issues (depression, anxiety, psychotic disorders)	
Substance abuse (alcohol, prescription, recreational drugs, tobacco)	
HIV/AIDS	
Other	

Provide details on your nuclear family, especially if there is any relevant clinical data that would be important to understand your family history. Please feel free to add as many relatives as needed to cover such instances.

FAMILY MEMBER	ALIVE OR DECEASED?	AGE AND HEALTH CONDITION (IF DECEASED, INDICATE DATE OF DEATH AND CAUSE OF DEATH)
Mother		
Father		
Child		
Sibling—male		
Sibling—female		
Maternal grandmother		
Maternal grandfather		
Paternal grandmother		
Paternal grandfather		

Add details about your extended family, especially if there is any relevant clinical data that would be important to understand your family history. Please feel free to add as many relatives as needed to cover such instances.

FAMILY MEMBER	ALIVE OR DECEASED?	AGE AND HEALTH CONDITION (IF DECEASED, INDICATE DATE OF DEATH AND CAUSE OF DEATH)
Maternal aunt		
Maternal uncle		
Maternal cousin		
Paternal aunt		
Paternal uncle		
Paternal cousin		

LIFESTYLE

Please answer the following questions to the best of your ability.

General Information

Marital status:

Do you have children?

Do you have grandchildren?

How close are your ties to your family and friends?

What is your occupation?

What are your hobbies?

Do you travel outside the country?

Do you use a seat belt?

Do you have a working smoke detector?

Do you have a working carbon monoxide detector?

Sleep

On an average, how many hours of restful sleep do you get per night?

How many hours of sleep do you think you need?

Do you suffer from insomnia, hypersomnia, or sleep apnea?

During the past month, what percent of the time would you say you wake up feeling fresh and fully rested?

Have there been any major changes in your sleep patterns in the last year?

Do you find it difficult to get out of bed in the morning?

Substance Use

How many servings of an alcoholic beverage (include type—beer, wine, etc.) do you consume in an average week?

Do you currently use tobacco? If yes, what type, for how long, and have you ever tried to quit?

Have you ever used any type of tobacco in the past? If yes, what type, for how long, and when did you quit?

Personal Assessment

The list below contains several traits that describe people. Select the answer that best describes you with the following responses: definitely not you (DNY), somewhat like you (SLY), much like you (MLY), or very much like you (VMLY).

Have a need to excel in mostly everything	____
Always rushed or pressed for time	____
Eat most meals too fast	____
Hard driven and competitive	____
Bossy and domineering	____

When you are very angry or upset about something, rate each response according to the likelihood of having the listed reaction. Rate with the following: not too likely, somewhat likely, or very likely.

REACTION	NOT TOO LIKELY, SOMEWHAT LIKELY, OR VERY LIKELY
Take a few breaths and talk it out	
Act like nothing is wrong or that nothing has happened	
Blame it on someone else (it's never your fault)	
Apologize even if you are right	
Take it out on someone else	
Talk it out with someone such as a friend or relative	
Get it out in the open (off your chest)	
Keep it to yourself	

On an average workday, please indicate (yes/no) if you generally feel the following. If you are a homemaker, refer to your household duties; if you are unemployed or retired, think back to your last position.

SYMPTOM	YES/NO
Often feel inadequate or unsure of your performance	
Often feel "stretched to the max" with your duties	
Often feel pressured or very pressed for time	
Often times feel like work follows you home	
In general, do you get upset if you have to wait for something?	

STRESS MANAGEMENT

Do you consider yourself to be under a great deal of stress?

From the list, select all the methods you use to relieve tension and/or stress:

LISTEN TO MUSIC/ PLAY MUSIC	SMOKE CIGARETTES/PIPE	SLEEP	WATCH TELEVISION
Cry	Throw things	Meditate	Blow up
Eat	Exercise or walk	Don't think about it	Work/housework
Do nothing	Turn to faith/pray	Take a drug	Go for a drive
Call a friend/ relative	Draw/paint/hobby	Have an alcoholic drink	Read
Other			

Mind and Emotions

Are you experiencing the listed symptom to a substantial or unusual degree?

SYMPTOM	YES/NO
Rapid mood swings	
Impatient, moody, nervous	
Lack of mental alertness	
Depression	
Anxiety/fear	
Lack of self-esteem	
Difficulty with memory, attention, or concentration	
Short attention span	
Personality changes	
Short temper/anger/irritability	
Excessive worrying	
Suicidal thoughts	
Confusion/poor comprehension	
Difficulty making decisions	
Restlessness, hyperactivity, or inability to relax	
Change in eating habits with depression	
Change in eating habits with stress or anxiety	
Change in eating habits with family or friends	
Apathy/lethargy	

You have reached the end of your Precision Health Questionnaire (PHQ). Great!

Remember to copy or scan this into your personal files; it is the start of owning your own record. In the future, you may add an update on a family member's health status or another new bit of diagnostic lab data on yourself. You will also want to bring your PHQ record to your doctor to share. Further you can use the PHQ as a point of comparison with the individuals in this book, and refer back to the chapters that address your specific health goals.

Finally, you may want to explore options beyond those available in my book. Our Web site KeepItUpTheBook.com will guide you in doing so. For example, should you obtain the metabolic and hormone tests recommended in Chapters 3 and 4, you might opt to enter your PHQ data and lab stats and then undergo an online Precision Medicine analysis. Welcome to your healthy future!

REFERENCES

INTRODUCTION

Allan, CA, BJG Strauss, HG Burger, EA Forbes, RI McLachlan. "Testosterone therapy prevents gain in visceral adipose tissue and loss of skeletal muscle in non-obese aging men." *Journal of Clinical Endocrinology and Metabolism* 93.1 (2008): 139–46.

Bonora, E, S Kiechi, A Mayr, G Zoppini, G Targher, RC Bonadonna, J Willeit. "High-normal HbA1C is a strong predictor of type 2 diabetes in the general population." *Diabetes Care* (2011). doi: 10.2337/dc10–1180.

Jankowska, EA, B Biel, J Majda, A Szklarska, M Lopuszanska, M Medras, SD Anker, W Banasiak, PA Poole-Wilson, P Ponikowski. "Anabolic deficiency in men with chronic heart failure." *Circulation* 114 (2006): 1829–37.

Matsumoto, A. "Andropause: Clinical implications of decline in serum testosterone levels with aging with men." *Journal of Gerontology* 57A.2 (2002): M76–M99.

Mayo Clinic. "Male menopause: Myth or reality." Mayo Foundation for Medical Education and Research, July 23, 2011. Accessed, April 19, 2013.

Mirnezami, R, J Nicholson, A Darzi. "Preparing for Precision Medicine." *New England Journal of Medicine* 366 (2012): 489–91.

Wehr, E, S Pilz, BO Boehm, W Marz, T Grammer, B Obermayer-Pietsch. "Low free testosterone is associated with heart failure mortality in older men referred for coronary angiography." *European Journal of Heart Failure* 13 (2011): 482–88.

CHAPTER 1

Aversa, A, R Bruzziches, D Francomano, M Natali, P Gareri, and G Spera. "Endothelial dysfunction and erectile dysfunction in the aging man." *Journal of Urology* 17 (2010): 38–47.

Comite FC, J. Baek. "Hormonal expression of androgen decline in aging men (ADAM)." Program: Abstracts—Orals, Featured Poster Presentations, and Posters. The Endocrine Society's 95th Annual Meeting and Expo. June 15, 2013.

Feldman, HA, C Longcope, CA Derby, CB Johannes, AB Araujo, AD Coviello, WJ Bremner, JB McKinlay. "Age trends in the level of serum testosterone and other hormones in middle-aged men: Longitudinal results from the Massachusetts Male Aging Study." *Journal of Clinical Endocrinology and Metabolism* 87.2 (2002): 589–98.

Inman, BA, JL St. Sauver, DJ Jacobson, ME McGree, A Nehra, MM Lieber, VL Roger, SJ Jacobsen. "A population-based, longitudinal study of erectile dysfunction and future coronary artery disease." *Mayo Clinic Proceedings* 84.2 (2009): 108–13.

Ridker, PM. "C-reactive protein. A simple test to help predict risk of heart attack and stroke." *Circulation*. 108 (2003): e81–5.

Shores, MM, NL Smith, CW Forsberg, BD Anawalt, and AM Matsumoto. "Testosterone treatment and mortality in men with low testosterone levels." *Journal of Clinical Endocrinology and Metabolism* (2012): n. page. April 19, 2013. http://www.ncbi.nlm.nih.gov/pubmed/22496507.

Takahashi, PY, PY Liu, PD Roebuck, A Iranmanesh, JD Veldhuis. "Graded inhibition of pulsatile luteinizing hormone secretion by a selective gonadotropin-releasing hormone (GnRH)-receptor antagonist in healthy men: Evidence that age attenuates hypothalamic GnRH outflow." *Journal of Clinical Endocrinology and Metabolism* 90.5 (2005): 2768–74.

Wald, M, M Miner, and A D. Seftel. "State of the art reviews: Male menopause: Fact or fiction?" *American Journal of Life Medicine* 2.2 (2008): n. page. Accessed http://ajl.sagepub.com/content/2/2/132.abstract.

CHAPTER 2

Comite, F, GB Cutler, WW Vale, J Rivier, DL Loriaux, WF Crowley. "Short-term treatment of idiopathic precocious puberty with a long-acting luteinizing hormone releasing hormone (LHRH) analog: A preliminary report." *New England Journal of Medicine* 305 (1981): 1546–50.

Corona, G, G Rastrelli, M Monami, A Guay, J Buvat, A Sforza, G Forti, E Mannucci, M Maggi. "Hypogonadism as a risk factor for cardiovascular mortality in men: A meta-analytic study." *European Journal of Endocrinology* 165 (2011): 687–701.

Dobrzycki, S, W Serwatka, S Nadlewski, J Korecki, R Jackowski, J Paruk, JR Ladny, T Hirnle. "An assessment of correlations between endogenous sex hormone levels and the extensiveness of coronary heart disease and the ejection fraction of the left ventricle in males." *J Med Invest*. 50 (2003): 162-69.

Ikeda, Y, K Aihara, T Sato, M Akaike, M Yoshizumi, Y Suzaki, et al. "Androgen receptor gene knockout male mice exhibit impaired cardiac growth and exacerbation of angiotensin II-induced cardiac fibrosis." *Journal of Biological Chemistry* 280.33 (2005): 29661–66. Accessed April 19, 2013.

Muller, M, DE Grobbee, I den Tonkelaar, SW Lamberts, and YT van der Schouw. "Endogenous sex hormones and metabolic syndrome in aging men."*Journal of Clinical Endocrinology and Metabolism* 90.5 (2005): 2618–23.

Srinivas-Shankar, U, SA Roberts, MJ Connolly, MDL O'Connell, JE Adams, JA Oldham, and FCW Wu. "Effects of testosterone on muscle strength, physical function, body composition, and quality of life in intermediate-frail and frail elderly men: A randomized, double-blind, placebo-controlled study." *Journal of Clinical Endocrinology and Metabolism* 95.2 (2010).

Sokolove, M. "For Derek Jeter, on His 37th Birthday." *New York Times Magazine*, June 23, 2011. Accessed June 23, 2013.

CHAPTER 3

American Diabetes Association. "Executive Summary: Standards of Medical Care in Diabetes." American Diabetes Association 33 (200): n. page. April 19,

2013. http://care.diabetesjournals.org/content/33/Supplement_1/S4.full

Boonen, S, D Vanderschueren, XG Cheng, G Verbeke, J Dequeker, P Geusens, P Broos, and R Bouillon. "Age-related (type II) femoral neck osteoporosis in men: Biochemical evidence for both hypovitaminosis D- and androgen deficiency-induced bone resorption." *Journal of Bone and Mineral Research* 12.12 (1997): 2119–26.

Centers for Disease Control and Prevention. "Diabetes Report Card 2012." Atlanta, GA: Centers for Disease Control and Prevention, US Department of Health and Human Services, 2012.

Cheng, P, B Neugaard, P Foulis, PR Conlin. "Hemoglobin A1C as a predictor of incident diabetes." *Diabetes Care* (2011) doi: 10.2337/dc10–0625.

Hanley, AJG, K Williams, A Festa, LE Wagenknecht, RB D'Agostino, Jr, J Kempf, B Zinman, SM Haffner. "Elevations in markers of liver injury and risk of type 2 diabetes." *Diabetes* 53 (2004): 2623–32.

Karikkinethm AC, M Canepa, P Elango, JB Strait, EG Lakatta, L Ferucci. "C-reactive protein as a predictor of intimal media thickness in a healthy community dwelling population of a broad age range." Poster session presented at Atherosclerosis, Inflammation, Biomarkers and Outcomes: What's New? ACC.13. 62nd Annual Scientific Session & Expo for Vascular Medicine. March 9, 2013, Expo North.

Libby, P. "Inflammation and cardiovascular disease mechanisms 1'2'3." *American Journal of Clinical Nutrition* 83.2 (2006): 456S–460S.

Lindsey, Cameron, MR Graham, TP Johnston, CG Kiroff, and A Freshley. "A clinical comparison of calculated versus direct measurement of low-density lipoprotein cholesterol level." *Pharmacotherapy: The Journal of Human Pharmacology and Drug Therapy* 24.2 (2004): 167–72.

Ridker, Danielson E, FA Fonseca, J Genest, AM Gotto Jr, JJ Kastelein, Koenig W, et al. "Rosuvastatin to prevent vascular events in men and women with elevated C-reactive protein." *New England Journal of Medicine* 359.21 (2009): 2195–2207.

Selvin, E, MW Steffes, H Zhu, K Matsushita, L Wagenknecht, J Pankow, J Coresh, FL Brancati. "Glycated hemoglobin, diabetes, and cardiovascular risk in nondiabetic adults" 362 (2010): 800–811.

Skretteberg, PT, I Grundvold, SE Kjeldsen, JE Erikssen, L Sandvik, K Liestol, G Erikssen, TR Pedersen, and J Bodegard. "HDL-cholesterol and prediction of coronary heart disease: Modified by physical fitness? A 28-year follow-up of apparently healthy men. *Atherosclerosis* 220.1 (2012): 250–56.

CHAPTER 4

http://www.ncbi.nlm.nih.gov/pubmed/1809076 Thyroid Function Tests.

Bartalena, L, F Bogazzi, and A Pinchera. "Thyroid function tests and diagnostic protocols for investigation of thyroid dysfunction." *Ann Ist Super Sanita* 27.3 (1991): 531–39.

Department of Defense. "Breast Cancer Research Program Fiscal Year 2000 Program Announcement." Department of Defense. http://cdmrp.army.mil/funding/pa/2000bcrpbaa1.pdf. Accessed June 6, 2013.

Finkel, DM, JL Phillips, and PJ Snyder. "Stimulation of spermatogenesis by gonadotropins in men with hypogonadotropic hypogonadism." *New England Journal of Medicine* 313 (1985): 379–81.

Greenwood, FC, J Landon, TCB Stamp. "The plasma sugar, free fatty acid, cortisol and growth hormone response to insulin. I. In control subjects." *Journal of Clinical Investigation* 45.4 (1966): 429–36.

Holick, Michael F. "Sunlight and vitamin D for bone health and prevention of autoimmune diseases, cancers, and cardiovascular disease." *American Journal of Clinical Nutrition* 80.6 (2004): 1678S–88S.

Norman, AW. "From vitamin D to hormone D: Fundamentals of the vitamin D endocrine system essential for good health." *American Journal of Clinical Nutrition* 88.2 (2008): 491S–99S. Accessed April 19, 2013.

Rudman, D, AG Feller, HS Nagraj, GA Gergans, PY Lalitha, AF Goldberg, RA Schlenker, L Cohn, IW Rudman, DE Mattson. "Effects of human growth hormone in men over 60 years old." *New England Journal of Medicine* 323 (July 1990): 1–6.

Traish, AM., B Abdallah, and G Yu. "Androgen deficiency and mitochondrial dysfunction: Implications for fatigue, muscle dysfunction, insulin resistance, diabetes, and cardiovascular disease." *Hormone Molecular Biology and Clinical* 8.1 (2011): 431–44. Accessed April 19, 2013.

Wallace, A. "C. Everett Koop, 96, former surgeon general with deep Philadelphia roots." *Philadelphia Inquirer* (2013). Accessed June 7, 2013.

Ziegler M. "Pediatric surgical training: An historic perspective, a formula for change." *Journal of Pediatric Surgery* 39.8 (2004): 1159–72.

CHAPTER 5

American Academy of Sleep Medicine. "American Academy of Sleep Medicine (AASM) manual for the scoring of sleep and associated events: rules, terminology and technical specifications." Westchester: American Academy of Sleep Medicine, 2007.

Cohen, S, D Janicki-Deverts, and GE Miller. "Psychological stress and disease." *Journal of the American Medical Association* 298.14 (2007): 1685–1687. Accessed April 19, 2013.

Dement, WC, and C Vaughan. *The Promise of Sleep: A Pioneer in Sleep Medicine Explores the Vital Connection Between Health, Happiness, and a Good Night's Sleep.* New York: Dell, 1999.

Dinneen, S, A Alzaid, J Miles, and R Rizza. "Metabolic effects of the nocturnal rise in cortisol on carbohydrate metabolism in normal humans." *Journal of Clinical Investigation* 92 (1993): 2283–90.

Fontana, L, JC Eagon, ME Trujillo, PE Scherer, and S Klein. "Visceral fat adipokine secretion is associated with systematic inflammation in obese humans." *Diabetes* 56.4 (2007): 1010–13. Accessed April 19, 2013.

Hadhazy, A. "Think twice: How the gut." *Scientific American,* February 12, 2010. Accessed April 19, 2013.

Huedo-Medina, TB, I Kirsch, J Middlemass, M Klonizakis, AN Siriwardena. "Effectiveness of non-benzodiazepine hypnotics in treatment of adult insomnia: Meta-analysis of data submitted to the food and drug administration." *BMJ* 345 (2012). Accessed June 6, 2013.

Leproult, R, and E Van Cauter. "Effect of 1 week of sleep restriction on testosterone levels in young healthy men." *Journal of the American Medical Association* 305.21 (2011): 2173–74. Accessed April 19, 2013.

Prinz, PN, KE Moe, EM Dulberg, LH Larsen, MV Vitiello, B Toivola, GR Merriam. "Higher plasma IGF-1 levels are associated with increase delta sleep in healthy older men." *J Gerontol A Biol Sci Med Sci* 50.4 (1995):M222–26.

Randell, D. "Decoding the science of sleep." *Wall Street Journal*, August 3, 2012.

Saaresranta, T, and O Polo. "Sleep-disordered breathing and hormones." *European Respiratory Journal* 22 (2003): 161–72.

Saul, S. "Sleep drugs found only mildly effective, but wildly popular." *New York Times*, October 23, 2007. Accessed June 7, 2013.

Sheehy, G. *Passages: Predictable Crises of Adult Life.* New York: Bantam, 1984.

Shenk, JW. "What Makes Us Happy?" *Atlantic Magazine*, June 1, 2009. Accessed June 4, 2013.

Smith, R, C Guilleminault, B Efron. "Sports, sleep, and circadian rhythms: Circadian rhythms and enhanced athletic performance in the National Football League." *Sleep* 20.5 (1997): 362–65. Accessed June 6, 2013.

St-Onge, M, M O'Keeffe, AL Roberts, A RoyChoudhury, B Laferrere. "Short sleep duration, glucose dysregulation and hormonal regulation of appetite in men and women." *Sleep* 35.11 (2012): 1503–10.

U.S. Department of Health and Human Services. "Alcohol and Sleep." National Institute on Alcohol and Abuse and Alcoholism, U.S. Department of Health and Human Services, n.d. Accessed April 19, 2013.

Valliant, G. *Triumphs of Experience: The Men of the Harvard Grant Study.* Cambridge, MA: Belknap Press, 2012.

CHAPTER 6

Ali, ST, RN Shaikh, N Ashfaqsiddiqi, and PQ Siddiqi. "Serum and urinary levels of pituitary-gonadal hormones in insulin-dependent and non-insulin-dependent diabetic males with and without neuropathy." *Archives of Andrology* 30.2 (1993): 117–23.

Araujo, AB, SA Hall, P Ganz, GR Chiu, RC Rosen, V Kupelian, TG Travison, et al. "Does erectile dysfunction contribute to cardiovascular disease risk prediction beyond the framingham risk score?" *Journal of the American College of Cardiology* 55.4 (2010): 350–56.

Campbell, S. "Promotional Spending for Prescription Drugs." Economic and Budget Issue Brief: Congressional Budget Office, 2009.

Chew, K, J Finn, B Stuckey, N Gibson, F Sanfilippo, A Bremner, et al. "Erectile dysfunction as a predictor for a subsequent atherosclerotic cardiovascular events: Findings from a linked-data study." *Journal of Sexual Medicine* 7.1 (2010): 192–202.

Hsieh, TC, AW Pastuszak, K Hwang, and LI Lipshultz. "Concomitant intramuscular human chorionic gonadotropin preserves spermatogenesis in men undergoing testosterone replacement therapy." *Journal of Urology* 189 (2013): 647–50.

Maurice, WL. "Chapter 9: Low sexual desire in women and men." *Sexual*

Medicine in Primary Care. Bloomington, IN: The Kinsey Institute for Research in Sex, Gender, and Reproduction, 160–61.

Mulligan, T, MF Frick, QC Zuraw, A Stemhagen, and C McWhirter. "Prevalence of hypogonadism in males aged at least 45 years: the HIM study."*International Journal of Clinical Practice* 60.7 (2006): 762–769.

Rogers, JH, I Goldstein, DE Kandzari, TS Köhler, CT Stinis, PJ Wagner, JJ Popma, et al. "Zotarolimus-eluting peripheral stents for the treatment of erectile dysfunction in subjects with suboptimal response to phosphodiesterase-5 inhibitors." *Journal of American Cardiology* 60.25 (2012): 2618–27.

Sternbach, H. "Age-associated testosterone decline in men: Clinical issues for psychiatry."*American Journal of Psychiatry* 155.10 (1998): 1310–18.

CHAPTER 7

Chiu, CJ, S Liu, WC Willett, TMS Wolever, JC Brand-Miller, AW Barclay, and A Taylor. "Informing food choices and health outcomes by use of the dietary glycemic index." *Nutrition Reviews* 69(4): 231–42.

Cunningham, JJ. "A reanalysis of the factors influencing basal metabolic rate in normal adults." *American Journal of Clinical Nutrition* 33.11 (1980): 2372–74. Accessed April 19, 2013.

Foster-Powell, K, SHA Holt, and JC Brand-Miller. "International table of glycemic index and glycemic load values: 2002." *American Journal of Clinical Nutrition* 76 (2002):5–56.

Gannon, MC, FQ Nuttall, A Saeed, K Jordan, and H Hoover. "An increase in dietary protein improves the blood glucose response in persons with type diabetes." *American Journal of Clinical Nutrition* 78.4 (2003): 734–41. Accessed April 19, 2013.

Gannon, MC, and FQ Nuttall. "Effect of high-protein, low-carbohydrate diet on blood glucose control in people with type 2 diabetes."*Diabetes* 53.9 (2004): 2375–82. Accessed April 19, 2013.

Harrison, M, DJ O'Gorman, N McCaffrey, MT Hamilton, TW Zderic, BP Carson, and NM Moyna. "Influence of acute exercise with and without carbohydrate replacement on postprandial lipid metabolism." *Journal of Applied Physiology* 106 (2009): 943–49.

Larsen, TM, et al. "Diets with high or low protein content and glycemic index for weight-loss maintenance." *New Engand Journal of Medicine* 363(22): 2102–13.

Ross, GW, RD Abbott, H Petrovitch, DM Morens, A Grandinetti, K Tung, et al. "Association of coffee and caffeine intake with the risk of Parkinson disease." *Journal of the American Medical Association* 283.20 (2000): 2674–79. Accessed April 19, 2013.

Signorile, J. *Bending the Aging Curve.* Champaign, IL: Human Kinetics, 2011.

Teta, J, and K Teta. "Hormonal Weight Loss." *Metabolic Effect.* http://shop .metaboliceffect.com/topic/39-exercise-science.aspx Accessed May 28, 2013.

CHAPTER 8

Brown, GA, MD Vukovich, RL Sharp, TA Reifenrath, KA Parsons, and DS King. "Effect of Oral DHEA on serum testosterone and adaptations to resistance training in young men." *Journal of Applied Physiology* 87.6 (1999): 2274–83. Accessed April 19, 2013.

Costill, DL, GP Dalsky, WJ Fink. "Effects of caffeine ingestion on metabolism and exercise performance." *Med Sci Sports* 10.3 (1978): 155–58.

Crozier, SJ, AG Preston, JW Hurst, MJ Payne, J Mann, L Hainly, and DL Miller. "Cacao seeds are a 'Super Fruit': A comparative analysis of various fruit powder and products." *Chemistry Central Journal* 5.5 (2011): n. page. Accessed April 19, 2013.

Fenech, M, C Aitken, and J Rinaldi. "Folate, vitamin B12, homocysteine status and DNA damage in young Australian adults." *Carcinogenesis* 19.7 (1998): 1163–71.

Fisher N, M Hughes, M Gerhard-Herman, and NK Hollenberg. "Flavanol-rich cocoa induces nitric-oxide-dependent vasodilation in healthy humans." *Journal of Hypertension* 21.12 (2003): 2281–86 (Art23).

Flakoll, PJ, T Judy, K Flinn, C Carr, S Flinn. "Postexercise protein supplementation improves health and muscle soreness during basic military training in marine recruits." *Journal of Applied Physiology* 96 (2004): 951–56.

Fotino, AD, AM Thompson-Paul, LA Bazzano. "Effect of coenzyme Q10 supplementation on heart failure: A meta-analysis." *American Journal of Clinical Nutrition* 97.2 (2013): 268–75.

Ignarro, LJ. "Nitric oxide: A unique endogenous signaling molecule in vascular biology." *Bioscience Reports* 19.2 (1999): 51–71.

Kim, LS, LJ Axelrod, P Howard, N Buratovich, and RF Waters. "Efficacy of methylsufonylmethane (MSM) in osteoarthritis pain of the knee: A pilot clinical trial."*Osteoarthritis and Cartilage* 14.3 (2006): 286–94. Accessed April 19, 2013.

Littaru, GP, and P Langsjoen. "Coenzyme Q10 and statins: Biochemical and clinical implications." *Mitochondrion* 7 (2007): S168–S174. Accessed April 19, 2013.

Mann, NJ, D Li, AJ Sinclair, NPB Dudman, XW Guo, GR Elsworth, AK Wilson, and FD Kelly. "The effect of diet on plasma homocysteine concentrations in healthy male subjects" *European Journal of Clinical Nutrition* 53 (1999): 895–99.

Mortensen, CoQ10 Heart Failure, 2013.

Steels, E, A Rao, and E Vitetta. "Physiological aspects of male libido enhanced by standardized trigonella foenum-graecum extract and mineral formulation." *Phytotherapy Research* 10.1002 (2011): n. page. Accessed April 19, 2013.

Trivedi, DP, R Doll, KT Khaw. "Effect of four monthly oral vitamin D3 (cholecalciferol) supplementation on fractures and mortality in men and women living in the community: Randomised double blind controlled trial." *BMJ* 326 (2003).

CHAPTER 9

Basaria, S, AD Coviello, TG Travison, TW Storer, WR Farwell, AM Jette, R Eder, et al. "Adverse events associated with testosterone administration." *New England Journal of Medicine* 363.2 (2010): 109–22.
http://informahealthcare.com/doi/abs/10.3109/13685538.2012.754008

Chung, C-C, Y Kao, Y Chen, Y Chen. "Androgen modulates cardiac fibrosis contributing to gender differences on heart failure." *Informa Healthcare* 16(1): 22–27.

Dunkel, T. "Vigor Quest." *New York Times Magazine.* January 15, 2010.

Elbornsson, M, G Gotherstrom, I Bosaeus, B Bengtsson, G Johannsson, and J Svensson. "Fifteen years of GH replacement improves body composition and cardiovascular risk factors." *European Journal of Endocrinology* 168 (2013) 745–53.

Espeland, MA, SR Rapp, SA Shumaker, R Brunner, JE Manson, BB Sherwin, J Hsia, et al. "Conjugated equine estrogens and global cognitive function in postmenopausal women: Women's health initiative memory study." *Journal of the American Medical Association* 291.24. (2004): 2959–68.

Huggins, C, RE Stevens, and C Hodges. "Studies on prostatic cancer II. The effects of castration on advanced carcinoma of the prostate gland." *Archives of Surgery.* 43.2 (1941): 209–23.

Manson, JE. "The role of personalized medicine in identifying appropriate candidates for menopausal estrogen therapy." *Metabolism* 62. Suppl 1. (2013): S15–19.

Manson, JE (moderator). "Presidential Symposium: Plenary Symposium #1: New findings from the Kronos Early Estrogen Prevention Study (KEEPS) Randomized Trial." Orlando, Florida: Program and abstracts of the North American Menopause Society 23rd Annual Meeting, October 3–6, 2012.

Miller, D. "HCG popular among steroid users: Substance also often prescribed for other conditions." MLB.com (2009). Accessed June 7, 2013.

Morgentaler, A, M Hult. "Testosterone therapy in men on active surveillance for prostate cancer" (abstract). American Urological Association: Annual Meeting, May 5, 2013.

Moller, N, and JOL Jorgensen. "Effects of growth hormone on glucose, lipid and protein metabolism in human subjects." *Endocrine Reviews* 30.2 (2009) 152–77.

Norris, J. "Are higher testosterone levels associated with greater heart risk?" University of California, San Francisco, August 3, 2010. http://www.ucsf.edu/news/2010/08/5999/testosterone-heart-risk-research-raise-concerns-about-testosterone-replacem Accessed April 19, 2013.

Rhoden, EL, and A Morgentaler, "Risk of testosterone replacement therapy and recommendations for monitoring." *New England Journal of Medicine* 350 (2005): 482–92.

Rossouw, JE, GL Anderson, RL Prentice, AZ LaCroix, C Kooperberg, ML Stefanick, RD Jackson, et al. "Risks and benefits of estrogen plus progestin in healthy postmenopausal women: Principal results from the women's health initiative randomized controlled trial." *Journal of the American Medical Association* 288.3 (2002): 321–33.

Saad, F, A Haider, G Dorox, A Traish. "Long-term treatment of hypogonadal men with testosterone produces substantial and sustained weight loss." *Obesity* (April 2013) doi: 10.1002/oby.20407 (accessed May 28, 2013).

Tsujimura, A, K Matsumiya, T Takao, Y Miyagawa, S Takada, M Koga, M Koga, et al. "Treatment with Human Chorionic Gonadotropin for PADAM: A preliminary report." *Aging Male: The Official Journal of the International Society for the Study of the Aging Male* 3.4 (2005): 175–79.

Yu, G, and AM Traish. "Induced testosterone deficiency: From clinical presentation of fatigue, erectile dysfunction and muscle atrophy to insulin resistance and diabetes." *Hormone Molecular Biology and Clinical Investigation* 8.1 (2011): 425–30.

CHAPTER 10

Arsenault, BJ, SM Boekholdt, GK Hovingh, CL Hyde, DA DeMicco, A Chatterjee, P Barter, P Deedwania, DD Waters, JC LaRosa, TR Pedersen, and JJP Kastelein. "The 719Arg variant of KIF6 and cardiovascular outcomes in statin-treated, stable coronary patients of the treating to new targets and incremental decrease in end points through aggressive lipid-lowering prospective studies." *Circ Cardiovasc Genet* 5 (2012): 51–57.

Bangen, KJ, A Beiser, L Delano-Wood, DA Nation, M Lamar, DJ Libon, MW Bondi, S Seshadri, PA Wolf, R Au. "ApoE genotype modifies the relationship between midlife vascular risk factors and later cognitive decline." *Journal of Stroke and Cerebrovascular Diseases* doi:10.1016/j.jstrokecerebrovasdis.2013.03.013.

Bittencourt, LK, JO Barentsz, LCD de Miranda, EL Gasparetto. "Prostate MRI: Diffusion-weighted imaging at 1.5T correlates better with prostatectomy Gleason grades than TRUS-guided biopsies in peripheral zone tumours." *European Radiology* 22.2 (2012): 468–75.

Deshmukh, HA, HM Colhoun, T Johnson, PM McKeigue, DJ Betteridge, PN Durrington, JH Fuller, S Livingstone, V Charlton-Menys, A Neil, N Poulter, P Sever, DC Shields, AV Stanton, A Chatterjee, C Hyde, RA Calle, DA DeMicco, S Trompet, I Postmus, I Ford, JW Jukema, M Caulfield, GA Hitman. "Genome-wide association study of genetic determinants of LDL-c response to atorvastatin therapy: Importance of Lp(a)." *Joural Lipid Research* 53 (2012): 1000–1011.

Danik, JS, DI Chasman, JG MacFadyen, F Nyberg, BJ Barratt, PM Ridker. "Lack of association between SLCO1B1 polymorphisms and clinical myalgia following rosuvastatin therapy" *American Heart Journal* 165.6 (2013): 1008–14.

Gomez, P, P Perez-Martinez, C Marin, A Camargo, EM Yubero-Serrano, A Garcia-Rios, F Rodriguez, J Delgado-Lista, F Perez-Jiminex, J Lopez-Miranda. "APOA1 and APOA4 gene polymorphisms influence the effects of dietary fat on LDL particle size and oxidation in healthy young adults." *Journal of Nutrition* 140 (2010):773–78.

Hastings, J, S Hennessy, SF Dinneen, and J Crowley. "High prevalence of abnormal glucose regulation in patients presenting for routine coronary angiography."

Myers, J, M Prakash, V Froelicher, D Dat, S Partington, JE Atwood. "Exercise capacity and mortality among men referred for exercise testing." *New Engand Journal of Medicine* 346(11): 793–801. Accessed May 18, 2013.

Nambi, V, E Boerwinkle, K Lawson, A Brautbar, L Chambless, N Franeschini, KE North, SS Virani, AR Folsom, CM Ballantyne. "The 9p21 genetic variant is additive to carotid intima media thickness and plaque in improving coronary heart disease risk prediction in white participants of the athersclerosis risk in communities (ARIC) study." *Atherosclerosis* 222.1 (2012): 135–37.

Sirota, JC, K McFann, G Targher, RJ Johnson, M Chonchol, DI Jalal. "Elevated serum uric acid levels are associated with non-alcoholic fatty liver disease independently of metabolic syndrome features in the United States: Liver ultrasound data from the National Health and Nutrition Examination Survey." *Metabolism* 62.3 (2013): 392–99.

van der Bijl, N, S Joemai, J Geleijns, JJ Bax, JD Schuijf, A de Roos, LJM Kroft. "Assessment of Agatston coronary artery calcium score using contrast-enhanced CT coronary angiography." *Journal of the American College of Radiology* 195 (2010): 1299–1305.

Vorlander, C, J Wolff, S Saalabian, RH Lienenluke, RA Wahl. "Real-time ultrasound elastography—a noninvasive diagnostic procedure for evaluating dominant thyroid nodules." *Langenback's Archives of Surgery* 395.7 (2010): 865–71.

Walter, KN, EJ Corwin, J Ulbrecht, LM Demers, JM Bennett, CA Whetzel, LC Klein. "Elevated thyroid stimulating hormone is associated with elevated cortisol in healthy young men and women." *Thyroid Research* 5.13 (2012).

Wilke, RA, LB Ramsey, SG Johnson, WD Maxwell, HL McLeod, D Voora, RM Krauss, DM Roden, Q Feng, RM Cooper-DeHoff, L Gong, TE Klein, M Wadelius, and M Niemi. "The clinical pharmacogenomics implementation consortium: CPIC guideline for SLCO1B1 and simvastatin-induced myopathy." *Clinical Pharmacology and Therapeutics* 92 (2012): 112–17.

CHAPTER 11

Bots, ML, AW Hoes, PJ Koudstaal, A Hofman, and DE Grobbee. "Common carotid intima-media thickness and risk of stroke and myocardial infarction."*Circulation* 96 (1997): 1432–37. Accessed April 19, 2013.

Kley, HK, T Deselaers, H Peerenboom, and HL Kruskemper. "Enhanced conversion of androstenedione to estrogens in obese males."*Journal of Clinical Endocrinology and Metabolism* 51.5 (1980): 1128–32. Accessed April 19, 2013.

Marks, LS, DL Hess, FJ Dorey, M Luz Macairan, PB Cruz Santos, and VE Tyler. "Tissue effects of saw palmetto and finasteride: Use of biopsy core for in situ quantification of prostatic androgens." *Urology* 57.5 (2001): 999–1005. Accessed April 19, 2013.

McGee, R. "Help Me Help You: Peyton Manning's Pursuit of Perfection Influences His New Teammates." ESPN.com. http://espn.go.com/nfl/story/_/id/8287028/peyton-manning-pursuit-perfection-influences-denver-broncos-espn-magazine Accessed August 25, 2012.

Ridker, PM, A Pradhan, JG MacFadyen, P Libby, RJ Glynn. "Cardiovascular benefits and diabetes risks of statin therapy in primary prevention: An analysis from the JUPITER trial." *Lancet* 380.9841 (2012): 565–71.

Verges, B, E Florentin, S Baillot-Rudoni, J Petit, M Brindisi, J Pais de Barros, et al. "Rosuvastatin 20 mg restores normal HDL-apoA-I kinectics in type 2 diabetes."*Journal of Lipid Research* 50.6 (2009): 1209–15. Accessed April 19, 2013.

Williams, D. "Meet the 49ers' Archenemy: Freddy P. Soft." ESPN.com. http://espn.go.com/blog/playbook/fandom/post/_/id/12862/meet-the-49ers-arch-enemy-freddy-p-soft Accessed October 12, 2012.

Yeh, ETH, and JT Willerson. "Coming of age of c-reactive protein, using inflammation markers in cardiology." *Circulation* 107 (2003): 370–71. Accessed April 19, 2013.

CHAPTER 12

Blackburn, EH. "Switching and signaling at the telomere." *Cell* 106.6 (2001): 661–73. Accessed April 19, 2013.

Brant, L, S Barreto, VM Passos, A Ribeiro. "Reproducibility of peripheral arterial tonometry for the assessment of endothelial function in adults." Poster presented at Markers to Assess Peripheral and Carotid Artery Disease: Rapid Advances. ACC.13. 62nd Annual Scientific Session and Expo for Vascular Medicine, March 11, 2013. Expo North.

Buettner, D. "The Island Where People Forget to Die." *New York Times Magazine*, October 24, 2012. Accessed June 4, 2013.

Chu, Louise, and J Buning. "OME 2013 yields pilot proposals to advance precision medicine." http://www.ucsf.edu/news/2013/05/105706/ome -2013-yields-pilot-proposals-advance-precision-medicine. Accessed May 6, 2013.

ENCODE Project Consortium. "An Integrated Encyclopedia of DNA Elements in the Human Genome." *Nature* 489.7414 (2012): 57–74.

Fonarow, GC, A Hernandez, D David, S Smith, KA LaBresh, and PC Deedwania. "Lipid levels in patients hospitalized with coronary artery disease: An analysis of 136,905 hospitalizations in Get with the Guidelines."*American Heart Journal* 157.1 (2009): 111–17.

Gorner, P. "Lori Andrews: Genetics and Reproductive Rights Expert." *Chicago Tribune*, October 1999, n. page. Accessed April 19, 2013.

Hayflick, L. "The limited in vitro lifetime of human diploid cell strains." *Experimental Cell Research* 37.3 (1965): 614–36. Accessed April 19, 2013.

He, FJ, CA Nowson, M Lucas, and GA MacGregor. "Increased consumption of fruit and vegetables is related to a reduced risk of coronary heart disease: Meta-analysis of cohort studies." *Journal of Human Hypertension* 21 (2007): 717–28. Accessed April 19, 2013.

Kolata, G. "Bits of Mystery DNA, Far from 'Junk,' Play Crucial Role." *New York Times*, September 5 2012. Accessed April 30, 2013.

Miller, P. "A Thing or Two about Twins." *National Geographic*. January 2012. Accessed June 7, 2013.

Toward Precision Medicine: Building a Knowledge Network for Biomedical Research and a New Taxonomy of Disease. National Research Council Committee on a Framework for Development a New Taxonomy of Disease. Washington, DC: National Academies Press, 2011.

INDEX

Underscored page references indicate sidebars.